When Neurons Tell Stories

A Layman's Guide to the Neuroscience of

Mental Illness and Health

Erin Hawkes-Emiru

Library and Archives Canada Cataloguing in Publication

Title: When neurons tell stories : a layman's guide to the neuroscience of mental illness and
  health / by Erin Hawkes-Emiru.
Other titles: Layman's guide to the neuroscience of mental illness and health
Names: Hawkes-Emiru, Erin, 1979- author.
Description: Includes bibliographical references.
Identifiers: Canadiana 20210123494 | ISBN 9781927637388 (softcover)
Subjects: LCSH: Schizophrenia—Pathophysiology—Popular works. | LCSH: Neurosciences—Popular works. |
  LCSH: Schizophrenia—Popular works.
Classification: LCC RC514 .H38 2021 | DDC 616.89/807—dc23

Bridgeross Communications
Dundas, Ontario, Canada
ISBN 978-1-927637-38-8

Table of Contents

My Mind

If you did peer
Between my ears
What would appear
Are lush valleys
Where I pick the words
That you see here
There are tall trees
Filled with ideas
And clouds that float dreams
Snow covered mountain peaks
Supplying creeks that flow with thoughts
Through caves which store them all
Until I recall
The chosen ones
From in my head
Put them on paper
So they can be read

Waves

Brainwaves wash up on my mind's shore
I never quite know what's in store
Maybe they will bring good thoughts
Like so many times before
If they can make others happy
Please then bring me more
I will write them out
Perhaps creating folklore
They all come from my heart
Right from my inner core
Some tell stories
About the many costumes
I have wore

- **Miguel 2019**

Introduction Part 1

The Neuroscience I Love

I fell in love. It was the fall term of my third year of my undergraduate degree and I was taking *Introduction to Neuroscience* as an elective. With each class I took in this new subject, I was more and more hooked; at so many levels, the workings of the brain fascinated me. The new language, concepts, and theories of neuroanatomy and its neurochemistry leapt into my head, and I was enthralled: was I studying my own brain? Within the term, I had switched majors and now set out to finish a BSc in Biology and Chemistry, with a good measure of Psychology. (I'm dating myself here, given that there were then yet very few undergraduate programs in Neuroscience.) I earned my BSc in Halifax, Nova Scotia - at Mount Saint Vincent and Dalhousie Universities, a joint Honours program between these schools - and then completed an MSc in Neuroscience at the University of British Columbia in Vancouver. I've been the recipient of numerous prestigious awards and scholarships, including two Natural

Sciences and Engineering Research Council of Canada (NSERC) grants and a Michael Smith award. My papers were published in a variety of academic peer-reviewed journals in conjunction with my supervisors, colleagues, and fellow students. For several years, I attended and presented my research at the massive (35,000+ attendees) Society for Neuroscience conferences. I was accepted, and began, my PhD.

But things were not all rosy. I was struggling with a diagnosis of schizophrenia, and dealing with medications, hospitalizations, and symptoms that included cognitive complications. Finally, I admitted defeat, and withdrew from the doctoral program. The next day, I received notice of that Michael Smith award. I had to decline.

Yet now, with stable years upon me, I come back to that love sparked many years ago. I've delighted in my return to the journals of neuroscience, reading and pondering. I'm hoping to bring you on a tour of the neuroscience of schizophrenia and other related topics. The people who will bring this neuroscience to life are my clients, people who experience mental health and addiction challenges. Their stories form the backbone of this book. First, though, this Introduction will provide you with an overview of some basic neuroscience, to prepare you for the rest. I've tried to simplify things, but hopefully without compromising the beautiful complexity that is the human brain. Throughout the book, I've tended to put the more basic explanations in the text, with some more complicated or more specialized items in brackets. This introduction gets quite technical, but you can enjoy the book without worrying about these details too much. Take as much or as little as feels right for you.

The brain - that three-pound mass of gelatinous tissue inside your skull - boasts on the smaller side of 100 billion (that's 100,000,000,000!) neurons and about the same for "helper" cells (glial cells). Neurons vary in size, shape, and development but there are some basics to consider. First, the anatomy of a neuron: like any other cell in our bodies, the neuron has a body (soma) in which the DNA has its headquarters (nucleus) and has the machinery for running the neuron (organelles that do things such as make and move proteins). The neuron has input areas known as its *dendrites*, where other neurons "talk" to it. On the other end of the neuron, its output projection, the *axon*, "talks" to the neurons downstream. Typically (but not always) the end of the axon of one neuron communicates with the dendrites of other neurons.

For the love of a synapse

This "talking" leaves us at where my falling in love began: the *synapse*. Early in the history of modern neuroscience - which was not that long ago, just at the end of the 1800's - scientists believed that neurons were all physically connected, in a sort of web. Others thought otherwise and discovered the synapse: a small but significant physical gap between the stimulating neuron, also known as the *presynaptic neuron*, and the one receiving the stimulation, the *postsynaptic neuron*. It's like a castle surrounded by a moat: someone swimming across the moat is the

10

messenger that gets from the castle (presynaptic neuron) to the other side (postsynaptic neuron) of the moat. For that analogy, the swimming "messengers" are the neurotransmitters.

Neurotransmitters are chemical molecules that the presynaptic neurons release into the "moat" and that the postsynaptic neurons detect after those neurochemicals have "swum" across the synapse. You've likely heard of serotonin and dopamine, two common neurotransmitters. Once they've made it across the synapse, neurotransmitters attach to receptors on the postsynaptic neuron. These receptors, which also come in many kinds, are what translate the first neuron's activity into a cascade of biochemical events in the postsynaptic neuron. In other words, when neuron 1 is active, neurotransmitters "swim" this message to neuron 2, which then can itself become active, "swimming" a message to neuron 3, and so on.

That was simplistic - in terms of the neuroscience it's simple... but, I admit, understanding the synapse is far from simple. Nevertheless, let's go a bit deeper. It is not just a matter of neuron 1 activity leading directly to the activation of neuron 2, then 2 to 3, and so forth like a row of dominoes. Instead, each neuron does some math. Neurons have many, many synapses on their receptive dendrites - some as many as 200,000 per neuron, though some conservative estimates put the average at around a thousand synapses per neuron - which means a single human brain has well over a hundred trillion synapses! The goal at each synapse is for the first neuron to make the next neuron more or less active. But, each presynaptic neuron that is active is not powerful enough by itself to make a postsynaptic neuron active. An analogy might help here:

Think of a committee faced with a decision to make as a team. The issue is presented, discussed, and it is time to vote on the decision. *All in favour, raise your hand.* Some people vote for the proposal, some vote against it. The ratio of "for" to "against" varies tremendously depending on the topic, members of the committee, and environmental circumstances. If more people vote for the action than vote against it, the action is taken. It is an all-or-nothing event: either the proposal is accepted or it is rejected. Neurons do similar calculations every millisecond, with at times massive numbers of "voting" inputs. They are either tipped into being active ("for") or are made less likely to react ("against").

Now we need some chemistry to understand what, exactly, the neuron is adding up. At rest, neurons are more negatively-charged inside compared to outside. Also, the positive ions that are inside versus outside the neuron are different: there is more potassium inside, and more sodium outside. Neurons work hard at keeping this so (using a *sodium/potassium pump* that brings three sodium out for every two potassium they pump in, thus making that inside negative relative to the outside). But all electrochemical havoc breaks loose when the neurotransmitter receptors on the dendrites get molecules of neurotransmitter stuck on them in the synapse. Some receptors let in a rush of positive sodium ions, a "for" vote. A rush of potassium out or a flood of negatively charged ions (primarily chloride) into the neuron is an "against" vote. Every neuron gets up to thousands of "for" (EPSPs, or excitatory postsynaptic potentials, to be exact) and "against" (IPSPs, or inhibitory postsynaptic potentials) votes. Add up the votes, add up the positive and negative ions from many synapses, and all of a sudden, if there are enough "for" votes, a critical threshold is reached: *Go! Now! We've made our decision!*

This decisive activity to "go" is referred to as *firing an axon potential* and is, like passing a proposed bill, an all-or-nothing event. Once the threshold reaches its tipping point, there's no stopping it. Starting at the decision point (the *axon hillock*, the part of the neuron that transitions from the cell body into its axon), an electrochemical rush goes down that long "output" part of the neuron, the axon. That *axon potential* travels from cell body to axon, not the other way around. At that first section of the axon, the new positive charge inside the neuron triggers sodium "gates" (channels) to open: *Come on in, sodium! Bring in your positive charge!* This positivity opens the sodium "gates" of the next section of the axon, which causes more positivity which opens gates which causes… well, you get the picture. (The movement of potassium ions is responsible for the subsequent repolarization.)

Then, it all ends at the synapse (a.k.a. the synaptic cleft). There the action potential causes the neuron's neurotransmitters to be released into that synapse. The votes have been cast and the decision to fire an action potential has occurred in response to the myriad of signals the neuron has received. Action potential by committee. The neuron then has a moment of rest during which no number of "votes" can make it fire. It works hard to get more negative inside again (with the ion pumps, in addition to passive potassium channels triggered by the passing action potential), and thus ready to fire another axon potential, if the committee so votes.

I've had the opportunity to "see" a synapse, using a specialized (read: *expensive...* easily a million dollars) microscope, an electron-scanning microscope. It is beautiful. I saw bulbous sacs of neurotransmitters in the presynaptic neuron, free neurotransmitter molecules headed - "swimming" - across the synapse, and dense receptors with neurotransmitters docked on the postsynaptic side. *So cool,* the nerd in me thought, and I fell in love all over again. As I noted earlier, researchers have estimated that there are over a hundred trillion (100,000,000,000,000) synapses in the adult human brain. Every millisecond or so, the pattern of synaptic activity in our brains changes, forming the basis of our thoughts, feelings, and actions. That just amazes me. I am in awe.

Introducing the "moat swimmers"

The whole nervous system (including the four lobes or sections of the brain: the frontal, temporal, parietal, and occipital lobes) uses axon potentials as their one (binary) language, but this doesn't mean that all parts of the brain do the same thing. For starters, different neurons use different neurotransmitters, including ones that make the next neuron more likely to fire an axon potential, as well as others that make it more difficult for it to fire. Neurons that release the same neurotransmitter clump together in the brain to form visible structures. This is the brain's "grey matter" - the neurons' cell bodies and dendrites. I like to see that some of these even have a certain tint of colour that makes them stand out. (The substantia nigra means "black stuff," the nucleus ruber ("red") is pinkish, and the locus coeruleus translates to the "blue place.") The "clumps" connect together to form neurotransmitter systems that can sometimes bring together areas of the brain that are quite far away from each other. Let me introduce you to a few of the most important neurotransmitter systems, though I do go into more detail as the need arises throughout this book.

First, given the traditional emphasis in research on schizophrenia and *dopamine*, we will look at that neurotransmitter's realm first. Some of the dopamine neurons have really long axons that connect the cell bodies residing near the back base of the brain in the VTA (ventral tegmental area) all the way to their synapses in the prefrontal cortex (PFC) just behind your forehead (part of the mesocortical pathway). That prefrontal cortex is where many of our "executive" abilities reside: our abilities to pay attention, use our working memory, and inhibit actions we don't want to take. Other dopamine neurons, involved in the wanting (but not the liking - these are different, as we shall see in Chapter 5) of rewards, also start in the VTA but go to the midbrain striatum (via the mesolimbic pathway) that includes the amygdala. Then there's the black-hued substantia nigra in the midbrain; it too projects to the striatum, albeit to a different part (via the nigrostriatal pathway). Parkinson's disease, characterized by tremors, rigidity, and a marked slowing of movement (bradykinesia), is caused by dopamine neuron loss in this substantia nigra. Dopamine neurons also synapse in the amygdala (emotions), hippocampus (memory), cingulate cortex (motivation), and the olfactory bulb. (Did you know that people with schizophrenia often have troubles recognizing and naming smells?) Dysfunction in the dopamine system is believed to be the primary problem in schizophrenia, mostly because the antipsychotics that are useful in treating schizophrenia all strongly affect this neurotransmitter system.

You may have heard of another of the major neurotransmitters, *serotonin*. This "happiness" neurotransmitter regulates mood, appetite, sleep, learning, and memory - all of which are classically affected in depression. Serotonin cell bodies start in the raphe nucleus of the reticular formation in your brainstem, and they project to almost every part of the brain. Serotonin is involved in psychosis and the actions of antipsychotics, although not as prominently as the dopamine.

Norepinephrine, a.k.a. noradrenaline, starts out in the "blue place" (locus coeruleus), and when it gets started, all hell breaks loose. That is, norepinephrine gets the body ready to GO. Heart rate and blood pressure go up. Stored glucose gets up and goes to the muscles that the person will use when they either face the threat ("fight") or run from whatever could harm them ("flight"). The norepinephrined brain is alert, vigilant, attentive, and, understandably, anxious. This state is obviously opposite to that of sleeping; norepinephrine is lowest when we have dozed off. These two states are achieved by two complementary systems, the sympathetic and the parasympathetic nervous systems. Norepinephrine is the key player in the sympathetic nervous system (acetylcholine rules the sister system, the parasympathetic one; see below). It tells your body's organs to stop what they're doing and be ready to move: you are "pumped" (your heart increases the amount of blood it pumps) and "wide-eyed" (your pupils dilate).

Back in the brain, norepinephrine is similarly involved in arousal and alertness - all set for some action! Yet norepinephrine neurons are relatively rare in the brain; their locus coeruleus is quite tiny, harbouring only 15,000 (of our 100 billion) neurons! Yet these few neurons connect to nearly every major part of the brain, where they make us attentive and, consequently, better able to retrieve and put down memories. On the negative side, when you are extremely scared or in much pain, these neurons are highly active and may stress you further. But suppress these areas and you will find yourself deeply sedated.

Acetylcholine, or ACh, as we heard in passing, manages the parasympathetic nervous system. This one focuses on the zen, the "rest and digest" or "feed and breed" we do when we're not in a stressful situation. ACh was the first neurotransmitter to be identified. With our ACh, we focus our attention, remembering things relevant to the object of that attention; we find the motivation of rewards with our ACh. To do all this, ACh works hard in the cerebral cortex. That's the topmost, thin layer of our brains that does the lion's share of our thinking; it's the part that is all crumpled up and covers the inner parts of the brain. ACh also touches base with the hippocampus (memory hub). ACh receptors let sodium, potassium, and calcium (another positively charged ion) through; it is thus excitatory and votes "for" the firing of an action potential. While there are two types of ACh receptors (muscarinic and nicotinic) we will concern ourselves with the one associated with nicotine, in Chapter 7. ACh also works with the dopamine system helping us see what is salient and what we should do about that.

Glutamate and GABA (gamma amino-butyric acid) are also neurotransmitters that show up differently in the pathology of schizophrenia. Like yin and yang, glutamate is the brain's most common way to have a "pro" vote (an excitatory neurotransmitter) while GABA inhibits or votes "against" the activity of their downstream neurons. This can help control excitation from getting out of hand. To do that, GABA opens ion "gates" that generally let negatively charged chloride ions in and positively charged potassium out, though there are exceptions (e.g., during our early development GABA can be excitatory). Now with glutamate, it is all about excitation. I've left it to the last, but it is far from least; in fact, it is the most abundant neurotransmitter in our brains. It is used in our memory hub (hippocampus) and facilitates learning, as we shall see in Chapter 2. GABA and glutamate neurons reside in the cerebral cortex.

The psychiatric perspective

Using that cerebral cortex, I visualize my brain, the brains of my clients: brains belonging to people living with schizophrenia. Unmedicated, there are just too many or too few of these neurotransmitters around and we hear Voices, believe our delusions, and are paranoid. These are the "positive" symptoms of schizophrenia: experiences that are "added" to our lives, albeit to our detriment. Glutamate's work is thwarted (by a variety of mechanisms), giving us the "negative" symptoms: aspects of our lives that have "lost" something that "normal" people have. Our faces may fail to show our emotions (flat affect), we lose the happiness of happy times (anhedonia), and we care less about choices in life (avolition) - not to mention the glutamate-related cognitive deficits we must also deal with. When the cognitive task of paying attention lags, memory tasks can become challenging, too.

Psychiatry is traditionally centred on the positive symptoms of schizophrenia, and gives lesser concern and treatment to the negative and, especially, the cognitive features. For one, positive symptoms are easier, in our current medical model, to treat. Think of a carver with her wood or marble: how much easier it is to trim away the excess, the stuff that doesn't need to be there, than to try and add some part to it. Cutting off positive symptoms is similarly easier than trying to add something to compensate for what is lacking (negative symptoms). But is it really easier to stop a brain from hallucinating than to make its owner show more emotion on their face? Are we perhaps defining things by the current state of antipsychotic medications? Later we will consider why dopamine may not be the be-all-and-end-all in explaining schizophrenia. Likely, dopamine is simply one of many voting members of our brain's committee that brings on our schizophrenia.

All in all, we know a lot; we know so little; but the pursuit of understanding what the brain is doing when it goes awry is an intriguing one. The scientific committee has to make a decision based on countless peer-reviewed articles and books on how and why some of us - about 1% of the population - develop schizophrenia. It is no simple or easy task to go from synapse to neuron to brain to person. My university studies - all ten years of them - were firmly set amongst the synapses and neurons, but now, having worked at my current job in psychiatry for over seven years, I'm just as intrigued by the people I meet and get to know. *I wonder…what is going on in my clients' brains?* is what prompted me to ponder the possible neuroscience of their daily experiences. It prompted me to write this book.

Introduction Part 2

The Work I Love: What is ACT?

I never thought about work as a peer support worker (PSW), but, jobless, decided to put in an application. This was prompted by a fortuitous encounter with Wynn, an officer with the Vancouver Police Department who has a passion for mental health care. I had been sitting quietly in the corner at a British Columbia Schizophrenia Society (BCSS) event when Wynn approached. He had asked someone to introduce us, so that he could tell me about this PSW opening on a new mental health and addictions team. He had read my book (a memoir of my experiences with schizophrenia) and thought I'd be perfect for the peer support position. Wynn gave me the information, and then told me that he'd "open doors" for me. Indeed, he put in a good word - several good words, more like it - and I attended an interview after quickly researching both the position and what, exactly, an ACT team is.

The ACT team, or Assertive Community Treatment team, is a mental health and addictions team that takes on the clients no one else in "the system" feels they can "manage" (a word I despised when it was used in terms of my own mental health care, and I vowed not to use it in reference to how I interacted with my own clients; though I do hear it being used at times at ACT). The traditional mental health and addiction treatment teams have failed to engage and support these clients. They are generally "high service users" (high contact with hospitals and/or the judicial system); ACT has been shown to be cost-effective by reducing our clients' use of these emergency and judicial services. Consequently, we are charged with a very vulnerable and over-looked population, people living with (generally) both severe mental health diagnoses and significant substance use issues. Many of them live in Vancouver's Downtown EastSide (DTES) community, thought by many to be Canada's poorest postal code. Most of our clients have had periods of homelessness, or have spent time living in substandard SRO (single-room occupancy) hotel rooms. As such, we are considered a "low-barrier" service. Clients don't have to make it to office appointments; we go to them on outreach - to their communities, their homes, their hang-outs, or even the places they like to pan-handle. We look for them; we look out for them.

An ACT team is multidisciplinary: we have psychiatrists and nurses, social workers and occupational therapists; the four ACT teams in my building share two general practitioner physicians, and administrative staff. There are some other types of therapists, such as recreational and vocational, and concurrent disorder clinicians. Each team has a peer support worker, too, though only in a part-time capacity. Yet no matter the position, each team member contributes to the team's daily outreach. We are all encouraged to get to know as many clients on our respective teams as possible. This allows us to share the burden of our higher-need clients. In practice, certain clinicians gravitate toward certain clients and vice versa, which is appreciated by those clients who get overwhelmed with meeting, at one point or another, a team of 12 or so different workers.

Drugs, both ours and theirs

Most of our clients receive antipsychotic medication, and most of them take it in the form of a long-lasting "depo." Our nurses are kept busy with these intramuscular (IM) injections, administered every two to four weeks. (A new IM medication has recently come out, Trinza, which needs only to be given once every three months. Great for our clients who despise the IM injections; a bit creepy to me, in that once it's in, that's it, no way to change it for three long months.) This depends on the client and the regimen that keeps them well. Others take oral medication, particularly clozapine, an antipsychotic that is particularly effective when others have failed to "hold" the client. But clozapine does not come in an injectable. For those who need the oral clozapine, but would lose track of taking the tablets, we do DWI: daily witnessed ingestion. That is, every morning at 10:00am or night at 6:00pm, staff will drive to the clients' homes and bring them their medications, watching as they take the pills. Some clients, once used to the daily administration, can graduate to a local pharmacy, to get their DWI there by a pharmacist. A few move on to getting a week's worth at a time in a blister pack, and we check on this regularly.

We at ACT have a harm-reduction perspective regarding our clients' use of recreational drugs. Heroin, crystal meth, and crack cocaine are common substances many of our clients use regularly, as well as plenty of cannabis (which is, I will note, legal here in BC). We educate in hopes of saving lives: Don't use alone. Try a small test first. Know your source. After all, it is the height (will it climb yet higher? there seems to be no end) of the opioid epidemic, and we sadly and tragically lose clients to overdose all too often. We, staff, carry Narcan (naloxone), a drug that temporarily reverses an opioid overdose, and we train clients to use it too, leaving them with as many kits as they request. Most of the overdoses are due to fentanyl, a super-powerful opioid that readily kills. The scary thing is, fentanyl can be mixed into another drug unbeknownst to the buyer. It is increasingly found in non-opioid drugs such as meth or even cannabis. It is a dangerous time to be a street drug user.

Being assertive and supportive

Not every client is pleased with their assignment to our team, and we may get a "fuck off!" when we knock on their door. But, as our name indicates, we are "assertive" which means we are also persistent. Once the client gets the idea that we are not going away, they often turn to become tolerant of us, then accepting, then even appreciative of our visits. Some call our office, asking for a visit (though admittedly it is sometimes just because they are in hospital and desperately want an accompanied pass to have a smoke). Our outreach visits are all recorded on an calendar application on the computer, and during our hour-long morning meeting we assign each clinician to the client visits, after which we quickly discuss each client of the day so that all staff members are prepared. Visits may be short ("Hi, how are you?") or long, as we offer support in tasks such as going to get blood work done, or accompaniment to a medical appointment, or banking, or shopping.... Many visits are conducted in a local coffee shop; coffee is a valuable currency and buys us some time to find out how they are doing. For staff safety (either because of the client's unpredictability or due to an unsafe building), we usually go out in pairs. As the PSW, my role is slightly different, given that I tend to see the same few clients one-on-one, for longer visits. I have been able to forge good relationships with my clients, although a few of them see my visits as that of just another staff member.

The ACT teams operate by current standards of practice and all the current buzz-words are applicable here. If you were to take a look at our clients' care plans, you'd see that they are *strengths-focused*: almost the first thing on a plan is a description of the positive traits the client has. "Creative... independent... able to communicate needs... seeks out supports... caring towards others" are a few examples of those descriptions. Being *client-centered* means that we listen to the goals, small and large, of our clients and incorporate them into their care plans; we suggest other goals the client may not be able to articulate or recognize. For example, a client may not be leaning towards decreasing their drug use, but we will still hold a goal of treatment for them as we wait for the right time to encourage them along this path.

As we do all this, we have to remember that we are also *trauma-informed* in our practice. Often, we have read or heard about significantly distressing periods in our clients' histories, such as having been a young Indigenous child taken to residential school. Many of our clients have endured abuse, particularly sexual in nature. We must approach such topics as the client leads, and with utmost sensitivity so as not to re-traumatize them by bringing their past into their present. A practice that encourages us to involve a client's full personality, the positive people in their lives, and their interpersonal environment is known as *psycho-social rehabilitation*.

Schizophrenia by committee

We operate as a team, or committee if you will, and by our consensus (the psychiatrists having the weightier votes) we support the diagnosis of schizophrenia for many of our clients. Schizophrenia by committee. I want to note that in this book I deal mostly with clients whose diagnosis is one involving severe psychosis, such as schizophrenia or schizo-affective disorder. This was done mainly to keep the book a bit more focused. That said, nearly all of my clients do indeed have one of these two diagnoses. Also, my own mental health diagnosis is schizophrenia and this makes it easier for me to identify with, understand, and empathize with clients whose diagnosis is similar to my own. While this book is meant to be primarily about my clients, and not about my own struggles and victories in mental health, I do dip into my own experiences at times to highlight certain concepts or to round out a discussion. As a PSW, my job is to offer empathy and I cannot do that without sharing the common battles I've experienced. If you'd like to read more about my story, please refer to my memoir: *When Quietness Came: A Neuroscientist's Personal Journey with Schizophrenia* (Bridgeross Communications, 2012).

Now, may I present to you a group of individuals whose stories must be told.

Chapter 1

Can I Trust You? Oxytocin May Help

"I'm not lying to you!"

"I'm just being honest with you guys," my client, Glenn, says, again. "I'm telling you the truth about it; I'm not making it up."

"Yes, I know," I reply, with natural patience. "You're honest with me, and I trust that."

"But I'm not lying to you! My legs hurt so bad - I can't sleep, I can't sit - I'm not making this up! You guys aren't going to fire me, are you?" He hasn't heard me. I need to speak louder than his anxiety for him to actually take in what I say, and, more importantly, for him to trust me.

"I'm so glad you are honest with me, Glenn. Please hear what I'm saying: I believe you when you tell me something. I trust you. But I need something from you, too. I would like you to trust me when I say that I believe you. Can you do that?"

"I - I think so." And, over time, he did.

Trust was not something that came easily to Glenn. In and out of psychiatric hospitals since a young teenager, Glenn has been traumatized and betrayed over and over again. Whom could he trust? The people that sent him there? The psychiatrists who glanced over his chart and with little thought prescribed seclusion, restraints, and forced injections without asking *why* Glenn self-harmed repeatedly? The callous nurses who laughed at his needs: at him stripped, shivering, and without compassion, locked in the cell-like room they for some awful reason called the Quiet Room? These years of abuse, cloaked as treatment, have deeply hurt Glenn. He tips noticeably into PTSD (post-traumatic stress disorder) and OCD (obsessive compulsive disorder), battling multiple, daily waves of anxiety that he tries to medicate away with his prn's (as-needed medication) of clonazepam. Sleep is no escape: the memories invade his dreams, turning into true nightmares. "I dream that I die... I see my own death," he says with tears. He is fearful and jumpy, stressed and anxious.

As Glenn experiences anxious thoughts and feelings, nightmares and shallow-breath panic, his brain/body's system for dealing with fear and stress is sensitized and therefore repeatedly overwhelmed. My first thought was that his *hypothalamic-pituitary-adrenal axis*, kindly referred to as the HPA axis, is in overdrive, given that our brains activate this axis when stressed. The HPA axis uses a cascade of hormonal messengers to ultimately get our circulating cortisol up and running to help us deal with the presenting stressor. In Glenn's hypothalamus, which is located centrally in his brain (under his thalamus), a message is passed on to his pituitary gland (also in his brain, just below his hypothalamus) and finally reaches his adrenal glands, which are a pair of conical organs on top of his kidneys. From Glenn's hypothalamus to the pituitary (via CRH, or corticotropin-releasing hormone) and from his pituitary to his adrenal glands (via ACTH, or adrenocorticotropic hormone), these signals culminate in the outer parts (cortex) of his adrenal glands: they release the cortisol. This "stress hormone" then gives feedback to the pituitary and hypothalamus: *Stop sending the signal! We have enough cortisol, thanks!*

As I noted above, Glenn is chronically anxious in a way that made me wonder if he is dealing with a hyperactive HPA axis producing too much of that cortisol, or is somehow biochemically more sensitive. We could test his urine or saliva (showing short-term cortisol levels) or his hair (for the same; it stays there longer) for cortisol, or measure the levels of the hormonal signals sent out by the pituitary and the hypothalamus. We haven't, but I don't doubt that Glenn is suffering from some form of maladaptive HPA axis activity. Perhaps Glenn's lifetime of emotional and physical stressors has sensitized one or more of the players in this hormonal system. In a large and comprehensive review[1] researchers found any number of relationships between the HPA axis functioning and PTSD: some hormone levels are up for people with PTSD, some are down, some are indistinguishable from control groups. Maybe feedback is not working as it should?[2]

---

[1] de Kloet et al. 2006

[2] Daskalakis 2015

While we are helping Glenn to reduce his anxiety with consistent support, counselling, and meditation, Glenn also relies on the three clonazepam pills he takes a day. This medication - a benzodiazepine or "benzo" - is one that increases activity in the brain's main source of inhibition, the GABA system. One system inhibited by GABA is the HPA axis, starting in the hypothalamus: GABA reduces the levels of CRH sent to Glenn's pituitary, which means a weaker signal is then sent to the adrenals. There, the take-home message is that less signal means less cortisol. Furthermore, clonazepam blunts the sensitivity of the adrenal glands directly. Glenn's cortisol regulation is thus hit twice. Little wonder he finds them helpful.

Glenn's norepinephrine circuits are also likely on fire, grabbing him up out of rest into heightened alertness quickly, via his sympathetic nervous system. It is the brain's way of getting the body physically ready to deal with a stressor, and norepinephrine release from the inner (medulla) adrenal glands is prompted by cortisol: *Hey, I need some help with this stressor!* Norepinephrine also affects the activity of the hypothalamus, which can then - again - alter the response of the HPA axis. Like almost any biological process, there are negatives to all this activity. In the hippocampus, for example, a long-term stress-evoked norepinephrine overload can destroy synapses or even make neurons die off.[3] Put simply and bluntly, stress can cause physical brain damage.

---

[3] Sapolsky 2000

The sirens are not for you

Glenn and I walk to the local Starbucks, as is our custom, and it is not unusual for an ambulance or police car to speed past, sirens filling our ears. A stressful sound for anyone; abruptly , Glenn stops in his tracks. I see on his face the terror that he feels rising in him. Schizophrenia's egocentricity combines with his memories of siren-blaring vehicles and forced trips to the locked psych ward; his anxiety hits him full force as his HPA axis quickly readies his brain and body to respond to this stressor. "They're not coming for you, Glenn. You're safe. You're with me right now, and you do not need to go to the hospital." Glenn looks at me as I say this, and, over time, the trauma reaction begins to dissipate. I try to redirect him: "These ambulances are racing to help someone," I explain. I redirect again: "They're doing a good thing."

Personally, I may be able to handle the sirens, but even I still feel the fear Glenn knows when we cross paths with a uniformed police officer, ambulance attendant, or security guard. We both feel our stomachs drop as our respective HPA axes and norepinephrine systems engage; we are scared and want to run away or hide. I'm at work, though, on an outreach visit with Glenn, and so it is up to me to gather my wits about me and help Glenn conquer these fears. I cannot call them unfounded - we both have been hand-cuffed away to the hospital without us understanding what we'd done "wrong" - but I can tell him that right now, they are not there to take him (or me) to the hospital.

It was with great pride that Glenn moved

slowly, steadily, past his deep-seated fears of being re-hospitalized. I knew he'd found some peace when once (at Starbucks again! A weekly coffee gives us so much to work on.) Glenn said, "I like your uniform pants." He was complimenting a uniformed man on his navy-blue pants, the ones with the stripe down the side of the leg. The officer looked a bit bewildered at the comment, but I could clearly see Glenn's own pride in his beaming smile. Glenn was getting his psychiatric stability through his own efforts, and well deserved that pride.

Glenn has more to be proud of, because he has literally turned his whole life around in the past years. This month, he will celebrate his nine years clean from crack cocaine. He stopped smoking cigarettes a few years ago. He no longer carves his intense fears and powerlessness into the soft skin of his forearms, and has put an end to swallowing dangerous foreign objects. He has been heavily supported through these challenges, but it has ultimately been Glenn's own voice and power that have solidified these changes and allowed him to develop a life of mental wellness. Yet, something still gathers up his neural circuits and bathes them in neurochemical anxieties. What other neural molecules might be at play in Glenn's brain?

Would oxytocin help?

Perhaps… could we blame it on an insufficiency of oxytocin? It's a peptide hormone known fondly as the "love" or "cuddle" hormone because it promotes bonding between new parents and their infant, and is associated with physical affection (such as from your mate). In other words, oxytocin thrives in and drives trust-based relationships. Oxytocin has also been shown to influence other brain systems, such as that of dopamine, a rewarding "happy" neurotransmitter (to oversimplify); oxytocin promotes belief, empathy, and trust. Glenn's past - his time in hospital, where his care was severely lacking in oxytocin-boosting interactions - may have damaged his brain's ability to produce or respond to oxytocin. Perhaps this affected his biochemical prompts to feel cared for and to venture interpersonal trust.

Then, there are, as mentioned, the nightmares. Glenn's PTSD spills into his dreams every night, wherein he is re-traumatized by replays of his hospitalizations and worse. These nightmares are so frequent and so intense that he dreads going to sleep at night. He dreams that he is left in that isolation room, naked and freezing, while staff laugh maliciously at him. He is powerless there, and so vulnerable. There is no trusted figure, no one to offer empathy. Glenn's need for social connection is mocked in his dreams, which is notable in that such social stress could have activated his HPA axis, flooding his brain and body further with stressed-out cortisol.

If only - maybe? - Glenn had had recourse to some much-needed oxytocin. This hormone can suppress the HPA axis,[4] keeping the brain and body safe from skyrocketing and persistent levels of cortisol. Oxytocin levels rise after psychological stress,

---

[4] Neumann et al. 2018

presumably an attempt to inhibit the harmful consequences of a sustained HPA reaction. As stress peaks, as measured by the level of circulating cortisol, oxytocin also reaches a high. Oxytocin therefore can be seen as a protective factor, even in the face of chronic stress such as that which Glenn has experienced. Glenn may have insufficient oxytocin reserves, or his brain may have difficulties utilizing what is available, due to his past of chronic stress. If so, I wonder if the progress he has made relates to having been, and continuing to be, better supported socially. Does he receive oxytocin boosts from his peer support visits with me, and in his positive interactions with his sister? Research suggests this could be the case for some.[5]

When Glenn gets overcome with anxiety, he would need more than a boost of natural oxytocin, and for this he turns first not to people but to prn's (*pro re nata*, his "take as needed" doses). Perhaps he needs these clonazepam pills to subdue his nervous system in order to get it into a state where his endogenous oxytocin can do its work. He may often be too anxious for the natural anxiolytic powers of oxytocin; he might be experiencing cortisol-mediated stress that his natural oxytocin cannot seem to buffer. Interestingly, oxytocin can target the same GABA neurons as clonazepam does: they both enhance inhibition in the brain. On a behavioural level, oxytocin helps us pick up on the social cues that aid in our pursuit of the oxytocin-boosting social interactions. Glenn has established relationships with

---

[5] Neumann et al. 2018

several members of the ACT team. Maybe in time, he will be able to extract more oxytocin from these interpersonal connections, and need fewer prn's.

While some targeted counselling could help Glenn work through the issues behind his anxieties, I wonder what a nasal spray of oxytocin every night before sleep would do for him. The hormone itself might promote sweeter dreams, but I think that a significant placebo effect could arise as well, compounding the benefit. I wish there were more relevant studies in the literature to guide our team's approach in this situation. A PubMed search for "oxytocin" and "nightmare" yields only two studies, neither of which looks related to the search criteria. But if oxytocin manages stress and anxiety while you are awake (682 studies appear with those subject searches), surely it could do so in sleep too.

To extend the idea: why not go around and give every client a nasal spritz of oxytocin? The product is indeed available - even on Amazon (sometimes)! And with good reviews to boot... though it is not for sale on the Canadian site. There are studies that have found intranasal oxytocin to promote trust, thereby opening the participants to the oxytocin-boosting benefits of trust-based social interactions.[6] The oxytocin can prompt people to become more able to accept and use social risks for their benefit. (It has been used to treat autism-spectrum disorders, too.)

But as with most things in life, there is a dark side to oxytocin. The trust that oxytocin promotes will

[6] Van IJzendoorn and Bakermans-Kranenburg 2012

be selective: as we each define our "in-group" it follows that this defines many as the "out-group" and may engender favouritism at best and xenophobia at worst. Oxytocin may cause gloating (*My team won over your team!*) and promote lies that serve the in-group. Research (such as the well-designed double-blind, placebo-controlled study[7] that found this) also found that oxytocin does not induce self-serving dishonesty. Glenn certainly fits this profile. He has made a commitment to being an honest person, and asserts so frequently, as this chapter's entrance showed. He is trustworthy, not lying to serve his own purposes, though he speaks heavily and sadly of building staff who "play favourites" against him.

Trust

Trust is not always interpersonal; it can be intrapersonal as well, involving how much we trust our own bodies' abilities to cope with stress. Glenn, for example, seems to find it difficult to trust that his gut can handle what he consumes. He is in constant flux and anxiety over what to drink; he goes from beverage to beverage: juice, chocolate milk, water, sugar-free drinks from crystals, Gatorade... "It's too hard on my stomach," he says of one, then another, and another, then returning to the first again with claims of, "it's good for my stomach." True, his stomach is sensitized from years of swallowing foreign objects when he was unwell, but his inconsistencies suggest that there is a psychological

---

[7] Shalvi and De Dreu 2014

component, too. He seems unable to trust his body. The ever-looming "hard on my stomach" provokes Glenn's anxiety, thus releasing stress hormones, such as cortisol, that in turn can affect the neurochemistry of his psychological wellness. I wonder if, in his gut, oxytocin is involved; visceral sensory perception, including pain signals, is mediated by oxytocin there.[8] Less gut oxytocin, more pain signals?

Trust and mistrust are complicated social endeavours, and Glenn has displayed them in interesting terms. He claims mistrust in others, including members of our team, but then forms strong trust quickly. It seems that if there is a hurdle - a new person - there is fear, not trust; but, if they jump the hurdle once, the team member is quickly and strongly "in" Glenn's circle of trust. Eleanor joined our team about eight months ago, yet within a visit or two ("hurdle") she became one of his most trusted workers. He opened himself up, vulnerable, with very little to go on - but it stuck. So much so that Eleanor had to step back from always volunteering for Glenn's visits and biweekly assisted grocery shops. Glenn picked up on this, and panicked: "Is Eleanor mad at me? She didn't call me 'bud'!" He settled down again when Eleanor again picked up his visits - and called him "bud."

This has happened before, and, given the regular turnover of staff on our ACT team, will happen again. Glenn told me a few days ago that Eleanor told him that she is leaving the team in a few months. Glenn was devastated. I didn't have the heart

---

[8] Jenkins et al. 1984

to tell him that his counsellor, Natalie, is also leaving ACT soon. This pattern is not new (he has lost Nicola, Sascha, and Rhea as case managers) but it has nothing to do with Glenn personally... but I do know how you wonder about that, given that in the space of a few years, I had nine different case managers at my own mental health team. Glenn has fewer psychological and social networks than I, and I worry how he will cope.

I call or text Glenn weekly, at least, to confirm times or suggest to him to meet me somewhere - for blood work, for example, or grocery shopping or a haircut. "Hi, Glenn," I greet him on the phone in a positive tone of voice. "What's wrong?!" he replies, jumping to the conclusion that plans will fail and visits will be cancelled and he will be utterly abandoned. "I'll run away and you will never see me again!" he exclaims whenever moving him on from the ACT team to a regular community mental health team is raised as a possibility.

However, I know, from the past, what will likely happen at ACT: a new person; a new hurdle; and a new, intense trust. Glenn will still fear abandonment, but processing the loss of a favourite worker does strengthen his mental health, in that it shows him his ability to be stronger than the loss. It inspires courage and a feeling of: *I can do this. It's hard and scary and feels like everything will fall apart. But look - I'm doing it!* Glenn is indeed doing that: when I hear the fear in his voice when I call him, he is able to be directed back to his own strengths.

Glenn's fears and anxieties are obvious when we do bus training. At first, he was overcome with anxiety when I merely suggested he accompany me, after our visit, to *my* bus stop for *my* trip back to the ACT office. With repeated support, he has expanded his independence using a few select routes on his own and can, accompanied, face long commutes on crowded buses and Skytrains. Yet still, his HPA axis is in full-stress mode immediately and thoroughly, preventing him from hearing what I actually say when proposing new stops, even though I begin gently with encouragement to simply start to take note of the landmarks and signs.

"A couple of stops after we pass Langara [community college], they will announce 'Langara Skytrain Station.' See how 'Cambie' shows up on the sign? That's our stop." I say. "Soon, you will be able to meet me in front of the Skytrain. Not on the Skytrain; I know that that is too - "

"No! No! I can't go on the Skytrain by myself! No!"

"Listen to me, Glenn, please. Not *on* the Skytrain, in *front* of - "

"No, please don't ask me to go on that Skytrain by myself. I'll miss my stop and get lost and raped and killed!"

I ignored the catastrophizing for the moment, focusing on his listening. "Please, Glenn, listen to what I'm saying. To meet me outside it, *not* in or on it. Hear me," I paused, waiting for Glenn's full attention. "Can you hear what I've said?"

"What?"

"Can you trust me that I will not 'make' you do anything you are not ready for?"

"Just don't make me go on the Skytrain by

myself. It's too confusing. I'm not ready." Glenn was still fixated.

"I'm not."

"Oh."

"Just like the buses to LifeLabs for your blood work. I trust that you will let me know when you are ready. I'm not going to make you do something you can't do." My experiences with Glenn were that he grew best when encouraged but not pushed. I wanted him to feel and recognize his abilities, to be empowered by his role in the bus training. I wanted him to see how I trust him, so that he would be able to see how much he can trust himself.

Trust Games

There is a game researchers designed, though Glenn might question whether a "game" can be properly used to indicate circumstances that foster or hinder real-life trust. Aptly, though not creatively, baptized as "Trust Games," they are, as any research tool, about numbers and trials and permutations reviewed in a meta-analysis.[9] They are at times employed while the (trusting) subject lies still in a functional MRI scanner.

The game commences happily: the researcher gives you a sum of money, $20 if you are lucky. Your job is to share with another subject, anywhere from $0 to the full $20 - your choice. The other person playing the game with you decides how much they want to return the favour and give you money back. So let's say you gave them $10, a fair deal in your mind. The

---

[9] Johnson and Mislin 2011

catch is that they could sit back, take the $10, and end the game. After all, this makes them $10 richer than when the game started and why should they care about giving you back any money?

Actually, they should care, because they get a return on any investment they make in you. For example, if they give you $4 of the $10 you gave them, you both get $2 more. The game continues, with you investing and the other player (hopefully) reciprocating. Hmmm, you wonder - if I gave them $14 to begin with, would they have given me more back? If I invest more, they can reciprocate more! We both get richer! Maybe I should give them all my money!

That is true, but could just as well be foolhardy (they keep all my $20) as brilliant (they reinvest generously in me, to our mutual benefit). What determines both roles' actions is trust. First, the initial trust, indicative of how much you trust people generally; then, as the game continues back and forth, you get a sense of how much trust in this particular instance is reasonable. Does the other person tend to reinvest generously or does he keep most of it for himself? Is the trust mutual or misplaced?

Trust becomes defined by numbers (money accrued), which researchers like. Tracking the money earned or lost, they can see trends. They have, for example, found that the best plan for both is the "tit-for-tat" strategy,[10] with the initial investment being a generous one. It is fair - you give to them, they give to you (or, you both withhold). Of course,

---

[10] King-Casas et al. 2005

42

they are many other ways to play the game, and people with certain brain injuries[11] tend to play in a distinct manner. One would suspect that, given the difficulties with social cognition common among those with schizophrenia[12] people would play Trust Games differently. Indeed, these differences are consistent and, from a neuroscientific standpoint, very relevant.

People, such as Glenn or myself, who have schizophrenia share less initially ($3?), suggesting that we are, at baseline, less trusting of others. How much would Glenn invest? He doesn't trust many people, doubting, at least initially, whether a rewarding relationship could be established. He calls me repeatedly to check to make sure he can trust me when we make plans: Will I return his (social) investment? Will I recognize the "money" or social currency he stands to lose? Will I reciprocate with my currency (dependability, consistency, empathy)? Glenn worries, checks in (as I've said) repeatedly. He is trying to trust. At first, he only gambles with the time it takes to get a caramel iced coffee at Starbucks. Later, we plan shopping trips, haircuts, and appointments across the city to get his dentures fitted. We even made it to Horseshoe Bay to meet up with his sister for a day. Yes, Glenn still calls, still expects my calls to be dire cancellations, but he is taking the risks. Some days, I think he'd invest $18 in me, others $12 (notice my judgment that he has surpassed the $10; I am trusting that he trusts me). I do think that

---

[11] e.g., PFC; Moretto et al. 2013

[12] see Lee et al. 2004 for a review

we're slowly working on building a trusting relationship and that he can lean on. It's new for him, and I try very hard to be the trustworthy peer support worker he needs. "Don't fire me!" is to me a suggestion that he has "hired" me with a measure of trust.

But why should people with schizophrenia trust less? After all, it has been said that humans, not excluding those living with schizophrenia, are hard-wired to trust. That hard wiring appears to depend on the health and integrity of a critical brain region, the insula, so scientists have put people with insular damage into trust games.[13] Give such subjects $20 and they will keep most of it, but when the reciprocations have been stingy, they will in turn offer more money back. Isn't that contradictory? Think of it in terms of not understanding risky choices. If they keep $18, they run the risk of not getting the investment; if they continue with then offering more than is warranted, the risk is not getting generosity in return. Either way, they risk losing money. As noted above, this has been demonstrated in both people with insular damage, and people with schizophrenia. The insula has been documented to be both structurally and functionally impaired in people with schizophrenia.[14] Could Glenn's difficulties with trust be related to the integrity of his insula? More on the insula later on. It pops up regularly in the neuroscience of schizophrenia; it is an established and voting member of the committee that decides who

---

[13] Belfi et al. 2015

[14] Crespo-Facorro et al. 2000

will live with that disorder.

Chapter 2

Paying Attention to Salience

Trust must also be established in our own sensory systems. We arrive as infants, bombarded by new sights, sounds, smells, tastes, and touches. Some are familiar but now clearer, such as the sound of the newborn's mother's voice, and some seem instinctual, as when an infant uses scent to find his mother's nipple. Vision, the experts say, is fuzzy, underdeveloped. Yet no matter the sense, we *believe* what our sense organs are relaying. We take it as fact and at face value that these stimuli are real. Strange and novel, perhaps, but real. The stimulation may be supportive or not, but the experience is still regarded as true. For example, a baby may hear soft, soothing words, or harsh and loud shouting; the former experience leaves the infant feeling safe and the latter one, anxious, but they both assume that the sounds they hear are real, and will base their reactions on that assumption. Otherwise, why coo at a soft word or cry when you are shouted at?

That sense of reality is the foundation for the

infant's first psychological task, trust versus mistrust. This theory of psychological development was put forth by the child psychologist Erik Erikson. Can the infant rely on the sources of the sensory environment to the end that he will be taken care of? She is not thinking or reasoning, or weighing the pros and cons, but rather building an internal sense or intuition of her world. So, we have two foundations: one, that sensations are real; and two, trust or mistrust develops based on these sensations. Putting aside the complexity of the psychological development we undergo, what if that assumption goes awry? What if what we hear or see occurs without sound waves or photons?

That is hallucination. Hallucinations can occur for a variety of reasons, and though not every person who hallucinates has schizophrenia, most people with schizophrenia hallucinate. These are generally, but by no means exclusively, auditory and verbal: "Voices." You know that you sometimes can't see the owner of the Voice, but because our brains are so wired to believe that active auditory areas = auditory input from the outside world, we (and I include myself here, given my extensive history of hearing Voices) *feel* that they are real. No, not just *feel* it; we *know* it. We *trust* it. Again: we are programmed to base trust on the inborn assumption that perceptions are not only real, but that they are also salient. They stand out. As we will see, seeing salience is something we all live with, and it underlies the fundamentals of learning and memory. Salience detection and response is processed by a neural network in our brain that can go awry in diseases such as

47

schizophrenia.

Making meaning

Soon after my memoir was published in 2012, I was invited to my first interview - by phone, on live radio. I remember it clearly: my emotions (performance anxiety mixed with excitement) ensured that the memory would be well-entrenched. I was ready - breathe! - as I answered the call in my younger sister's childhood bedroom (I was at home, visiting). The first question was an easy one, the answer to which I could recite in my sleep. It was: "What is schizophrenia?"

I opened my mouth to say something psychiatric. After all, I had been a psychiatric patient for years, and had outlined my experiences of positive versus negative symptoms *ad nauseam* in my book. I was also qualified to speak on the neuroscientific correlates of schizophrenia. Of dopamine, perhaps, and the neuropharmacology of antipsychotics. At that moment, though, my careful preparations and natural intellect fell plumb out of my head. "Umm," I began uncertainly. Then this followed:

"It's, um, the, a disturbance of… meaning! Yes. Meaningfulness. You think something's really meaningful, when it isn't, or, uh, you don't put enough meaning on some things that you should. Like, the Deep Meaning. Yeah…." I trailed off. And this was live. Maddening. The host expertly guided me to other questions, and I managed to finish the interview. But *meaning*? What about hallucinations and delusions, paranoia and negative symptoms and cognitive challenges - the outline of schizophrenia in the DSM (the American Psychiatric Association's' "bible" for diagnosing mental disorders, otherwise known as the Diagnostic and Statistical Manual of Mental Disorders)?

It wasn't until several years later that I appreciated my "meaningful" answer, and only recently have I begun to discover that a small but evolutionary "old" brain area, the insula, appears to be particularly relevant when we are making meaning of our experiences. The insula (a.k.a. the insular cortex), is buried deep within the brain and encompasses three folds of the cerebral cortex. Its location - at the junction of the temporal, parietal, and frontal lobes, deep behind our ears - sets it up for many roles. The insula is divided primarily into front (anterior) and back (posterior) sections, each of which looks a bit different (structure) and acts a bit different (function) from each other.

The insula by no means works alone, but functions in tandem with many other brain structures, most notably the anterior cingulate cortex (ACC) and the prefrontal cortex (PFC). This network - insula, ACC, and PFC - is referred to as the *salience network* and is key in how humans recognize the meaning of, and ascribe meaning to, events, thoughts, feelings, people, and objects. That is, our salience network helps us to figure out what we should attend to (especially at those times when salience deviates from our expectations). Further, this salience network determines how our brains need to go about telling our bodies when and how to react. As we process meaning, it motivates us to choose certain behaviours over others. When all is well with our salience network, this is adaptive; when our salience network is not in line with reality, strange beliefs and behaviours may emerge.

These regions of the brain - the insula, ACC, and PFC - that are involved in the salience network are home to a very distinct and special class of neurons, the *von Economo neurons* (VENs). Their axons are large and long, and their dendritic trees bushy, in a horizontal manner. This suggests that they receive a multitude of inputs from neighbouring neurons (on their bushy dendritic trees), and that they transmit their signals quickly, efficiently, and with good fidelity down their impressive axons. This is thanks to our oligodendrocytes - a type of glial brain cells - which wrap a 20% protein / 80% fat insulation called myelin around axons; some axons, such as those of VENs, have more layers than others. This is similar to, but not exactly the same as, our insulation of wires for faster and more faithful electrical communication. VENs are therefore specialized. And special? How's this: besides the fact that they are found only in the salience network (insula, ACC, PFC), they are also present only in a select few mammals. Think big-brained, "smart" animals: great apes, monkeys and other primates, elephants, and cetaceans such as dolphins. That's it.

Somehow, and for some reason, VENs have evolved to help these very few species. When VENs were first identified in humans, a somewhat arrogant assumption prevailed: that we as homo sapiens alone were blessed with those big and beautiful VENs. That thought has gone by the wayside, but only to intensify our curiosity: Why VENs? Why only here and in these select species? Certainly other parts of our brains need faithful, fast information transfer. Why the salience network? I wonder if human brains utilize these "meaning" neurons to establish and sustain identifying and reacting to what is salient, which has undoubtedly played an important role in our species' evolutionary success. After all, attending to life-threatening situations is the ultimate in meaningfulness.

Then, for some reason, people who develop schizophrenia earlier on in life show a lower density of VENs in their ACC.[15] This may be simply due to the fact that people with schizophrenia have, on average, less grey matter (where synaptic connections are made) in their insula and ACC;[16] our insula is thinner, its cellular structure is compromised, and its protein expression is abnormal.[17] Over time, starting before our first psychotic break and continuing as the disease becomes chronic,[18] this reduction in volume of the grey matter of the insula suggests that this may mean our salience network has a harder time processing meaning. My clients or I may feel that something - an advertisement, a photo, a passer-by - has become salient and we are driven to figuring out why. A detail is magnified; is the insula firing wildly, without normal constraint? *Importance! Salience! Pay attention!* My insula may be quiet as I wait for my client to return to me after they experience a

---

[15] Brune et al. 2010

[16] Goodkind et al. 2015

[17] Korey and Tregellas 2010

[18] ibid.

captivating salience, though I sometimes find their utter focus salient, too.

People with damage to their insula resemble, in some ways, those of us with schizophrenia.[19] Given the current emphasis on dopamine in the etiology of schizophrenia, it is not surprising that the insula is dense with dopamine receptors,[20] and accepts dopamine signals from elsewhere.[21]

The long and impressive track record of medications that impact the dopamine system throughout the brain (that is, conventional antipsychotics) suggests that this neurotransmitter system is involved in psychosis generally and in its disordered meaning-making specifically. In our current era, we rely almost exclusively on these medications as treatment for schizophrenia. There appears to be a real and substantial correlation between decreasing dopamine's activity and alleviating the symptoms of psychosis, as well as evidence that dopamine antagonists, such as our antipsychotics, "dampen" the salience of things.[22] But with these medications, are we actually aiming at the real target? Or, could some other system be leading the dopamine system on? This very well may be the case, and this role may be played by a different neurotransmitter, glutamate. After all, in many places where you find the release of dopamine, there too are glutamate receptors.[23]

---

[19] Korey and Tregellas 2010
[20] Hurd 2001
[21] Gaspar 1989
[22] Kapur 2003
[23] Javitt 2010

Glutamate is so exciting!

Glutamate is an *excitatory* neurotransmitter, meaning that when it is sitting in its receptors, it "votes" to promote the activity of its postsynaptic neurons. An "excited" or "pro vote" message to that postsynaptic neuron makes it more likely to also be active too, sending a message (action potential) down to its connections. To achieve this activation, glutamate acts like many other neurotransmitters and adheres to its receptors in a way that changes their structure (opening like a gate) and function (charged particles - ions - enter and/or leave the neuron through the gate).

Glutamate receptors may be simple that way, or more complex. Many glutamate receptors (e.g., AMPA) only need the glutamate to open them up. But then there are the complex glutamate receptors, ones with which I was completely enamoured during my last year of my BSc. These receptors, the NMDA (N-methyl-D-aspartate) ones, do have the "opening of a gate" action, but glutamate alone cannot make it open up. In the middle of the gate, NMDA receptors have a molecule of magnesium, which effectively blocks ions from going in - even when glutamate is there. How do we get that magnesium out? After all, the NMDA receptors are useless as long as they are blocked, no matter how often glutamate tries to open them.

Well, alongside the NMDA receptors, the simple ones (e.g., AMPA again) get their glutamate and open right up, allowing a flow of ions. If these simple glutamate receptors remain stimulated long enough (if there are lots of neurotransmitter molecules available to do this), this lets in *sodium, sodium, and more sodium* until the whole area in the postsynaptic neuron is more strongly, positively, charged. (Potassium and calcium ions are also able to get through the AMPA gate.) Neuron #1 (presynaptic) is working very hard to get its message across. *Fire your axon potential signal now!* it screams at the (postsynaptic) Neuron #2 with the glutamate receptors.

If - and this is the exciting part! - this AMPA receptor-related change in charge inside the postsynaptic neuron is strong enough, this dislodges NMDA's magnesium. Then, all hell breaks loose as more and more sodium and potassium ions flood through the NMDA gates - and, these gates are large enough for even bulky calcium ions to get in... which, because they are more charged (2+, as opposed to sodium or potassium 1+) they *extra*-excite the postsynaptic neuron receiving this message. (Though too much of a glutamate good thing can cause neuron excitotoxicity, which is basically and literally getting excited to death.)

Since NMDA receptors require both glutamate (a ligand-gated channel) and a change in where the ions are (this requirement means it is also a voltage-gated channel), they are sometimes referred to as *coincidence detectors.* They react only when the presynaptic neurons *and* the postsynaptic neurons are active. Why did this excite me so much? And why do I write about this in a chapter on salience? In a nutshell, this NMDA receptor set-up is what lets our neural circuits - us! - remember. It is called Hebbian learning (after the esteemed Canadian neuroscientist, Donald Hebb, who introduced the concept in his 1949 book, *The Organization of Behaviour*). This theory was nicely summed up by Hebb himself as "neurons that fire together, wire together."

Let's consider a small network of two neurons, which we will call Alice (presynaptic) and Ben (postsynaptic... B comes after A in the alphabet. Believe me, it helps to name them something other than "Neuron 1" and "Neuron 2."). When Alice and Ben are simultaneously active ("fire together") their structure ("wire together") changes in ways (such as bringing more receptors to the synapse) that make Ben even more likely to respond to Alice - like the next time Alice dumps glutamate out in the synapse for Ben to pick up. Phew - got that? Basically, it means that changes in the function (firing action potentials) lead to changes in structure (receptor number and kind). Alice and Ben are now linked, and when Alice activates, she reliably excites Ben. (Neuroscientists call this neuronal learning LTP or long-term potentiation.) This, in essence, is memory.

So we've got learning and memory at the neuronal level, but what does it matter to us? In fact, it concerns us greatly, because if our neurons are lining up in connected Hebbian "webs," it means we have a system to detect coincidence and meaning. After all, we remember things that have happened together (especially when they are cause and effect) or that are particularly meaningful to us... though, we don't always get to consciously decide what is most meaningful! I'm sure we all have memories that seem useless or random, and we can all attest to having difficulty remembering things we put great effort into learning, only to fail to recall the material at a later date (exams, anyone?). As you finish reading this book, for example, you will retain seemingly random bits (the names Alice and Ben, perhaps?) and forget much of the rest (such as how NMDA receptors work?).

We therefore all know times when this glutamate system has failed us, but it is all the more apparent when we consider schizophrenia. The activity of that key player in coincidence and meaning, the NMDA receptor, has been shown by several avenues to be dysfunctional in schizophrenia. Drugs that influence glutamate neurons (such as ketamine, a drug used medically for anesthesia as well as recreationally, and the recreational drug PCP) can induce a state that resembles that of schizophrenia (psychosis, cognitive dysfunction, etc.). The underlying pathology induced by these drugs is also similar to those found in patients with schizophrenia. The glutamate drugs do this by interfering with NMDA receptor functioning: they effectively plug the gate.

Bear with me: one more thing about NMDA receptors and schizophrenia. Glycine, an amino acid, also needs to stick to the NMDA receptor for this receptor to function properly (glycine is a molecular modulator). We could offer the NMDA receptors more glycine directly (glycine, obviously, or some other molecule that fits in the glycine sweet spot, such as sarcosine) or indirectly (e.g., stop the glycine from being taken out of the synapse by its transporter) with a pill... always a pill, it seems. However, there has yet to be a glycine-oriented medication that is considered effective at safe doses: most require very high doses and therefore have significant side effects. Early studies from the 1990's to the early 2000's found that large (e.g., 60 g/day versus the 2 g/day that we normally get from our diet!) oral doses of just plain old glycine itself led to a reduction in negative symptoms in participants with schizophrenia. Participants in one study were lucky: these effects persisted at least eight weeks after the glycine was stopped.[24] This suggests glycine can have some sort of lasting impact on the NMDA receptor functioning and subsequent neuroplasticity. However, if you're taking glycine with the antipsychotic clozapine, you may find yourself with more negative symptoms than if you were on another antipsychotic and taking glycine.[25] A few of our clients would be in that boat, if we were offering glycine - which we're not.

Then, there's GABA

The release of glutamate is often kept in check by inhibitory GABA interneurons. Why? Wouldn't we just need excitation in our brains? Think again of our voting committee: if they all rushed to always vote "pro" based on limited information - *Yes, the defendant could have done it. He did know the victim, and that's enough evidence for us. Therefore, guilty! Off with his head!* - they would miss the "inhibition" of the "con" committee members who consider more nuances to the decision: *Wait. Slow down. Let's think*

---

[24] Heresco-Levy et al. 1999

[25] Evins et al. 2000

about this. Did the murderer's DNA match that found at the scene? Does he have an alibi? Motivation? The more we, the committee, think about this case, the more we realize that maybe he's innocent. We've "inhibited" a rushed, rash positive decision, likely for the better. Likewise, I'm sure we all can remember times when we've almost said an unkind word to a friend, but inhibited it and didn't say it… and in retrospect we are very glad we vetoed those mean words that would have damaged our relationship.

Thus: if some of our GABA neurons are silenced by schizophrenia, glutamate can abound unrestricted (uninhibited), which in turn causes dopamine levels to surge in key areas: a schizophrenic state. Perhaps with GABA's inhibition turned on low, glutamate neurons poke and prod the dopamine ones, suggesting that the "real" cause of schizophrenia is not dopamine but instead these systems (glutamate, GABA) that provoke dopamine dysfunction. What, we wonder, comes first in psychosis: dopamine or glutamate/GABA dysfunction? There are complex interactions between the three neurotransmitter systems, connections that are at times reciprocal. But, fundamentally, it appears that dopaminergic systems are directly under glutamate's control. Some researchers[26] suggest that the dopamine changes we see in schizophrenia are actually secondary to a dysfunctional glutamate system - which calls into question the theories of, and treatments for, schizophrenia based solely on dealing with too much dopamine activity. It makes me

---

[26] e.g., McGuire et al. 2008

wonder about the episodic psychosis that appears seemingly out of nowhere (i.e., while on a stable dose of medication) in some clients, such as Thomas. Is this a result of his antipsychotic medication dealing primarily with his dopamine levels, but not those of his GABA/glutamate system? With this glutamate theory in mind, will we soon see more drug pairings? *Here are your pink antipsychotic-dopamine pills, and your yellow antipsychotic-glutamate ones too.* Would this work?

Leaving the old, learning the new: NMDA habits?

Changes in the brains of those living with schizophrenia may thus be fundamentally connected to the glutamate system, particularly how its NMDA receptors function as that coincidence detector and, perhaps, ascriber of meaning and salience. Not active enough, and we forgo ascribing meaning to things that we really should see as salient; too active, and there is Deep Meaning everywhere. Both can be debilitating. Of the latter, Glenn finds many benign comments as meaning terribly bad things, and apologizes profusely at things outside his liabilities. It is a habit, born of trauma and is his automatic and subconscious way of protecting himself from psychological pain. He *knows* at a subconscious level that if he apologizes enough he may protect himself from harm. That deep *knowing* is difficult to change.

"I'm sorry, I'm sorry, so sorry for being a bad patient," he repeated after a bad reaction to a new medication.

"It's not your fault, Glenn."

"But I'm sorry for it!" He begins to cry, and his anxiety rises.

"Glenn," I say again softly. I ask him to stop walking and look me in the eye. He does. "It's not your fault. Not. Your. Fault. Please, say that to me: 'It's not my fault.'"

He has difficulty with this, but, wavering, he does it: "It's not my fault." We continue our visit, returning to this topic as often as he needs. I've been trying to help Glenn with his excessive apologizing. After beginning to work with him about five years ago, for the first while, I simply brought each *I'm sorry* to his consciousness - "What are you sorry about?" - and reminded him that it wasn't his fault. (The times something was his fault were very few and far between.) More recently, I've been pointing it out more explicitly. We explore reasons for his outlook that make him feel he has to apologize - his times of being told everything was his fault when his schizophrenia and drug use was not yet under control - and I'm emphasizing that he is not in those places anymore. He is safe with and cared for by ACT, and he doesn't have to apologize to us. This intervention is making a difference, I see, and I tell him. "I'm proud of you," I say, and I think it helps. He is realizing that he doesn't have to put excessive *meaning* into every comment others make and every behaviour he does. He is learning new habits: observable to me and, invisibly, in his NMDA circuits. The old LTP memory patterns were really entrenched, and it has taken a lot of the new "firing together" to create new "wiring together." Little by little, he is growing pathways of positivity and, as we've seen, trust; he is learning how to ascribe meaning normally.

The meaning of pain?

Moreover, Glenn no longer feels the need to self-harm. Behaviourally, he is in a safe place in his life, and deals with stressors by leaning on us, his ACT team. We keep in touch by phone and texting in between visits, which helps him. Like many people who self-harm, he used to try to mix up the signals, to feel physical pain in order to not deal with the more painful psychological distress. It is, as I too know, effective, and this sadly perpetuates it.

The meaning of the pain is radically different in self-harm than in accidental harm, and so is the experience of it. Here, in the insula, we see the separation of the front (anterior) and back (posterior) insula. The back part of the insula may think the two pains are the same because the exact same pain receptors are activated in both situations, while the front portion of the insula knows more of what is going on to make those pains very different. That is, if you go from back to front, you will see that engagement is increasingly complex, higher-order, and abstract. For example, the posterior insula will respond to simple thermal pain (e.g., burning your arm by stubbing out your cigarette on your skin), while the anterior insula one-ups this and reacts to the *meaning* of the pain: *I'm a bad person who deserves this pain.* It deals with how we evaluate concurrent emotions, as well as empathic pain. The insula itself also doesn't discriminate between physical pain and psychological pain. The "sting of rejection" and the "sting of a bee" both register in the insula and, interestingly, both can be relieved by painkillers such as Tylenol. I wonder: would Glenn's painful nightmares of rejection and psychological torment be even worse if he didn't take his four Tylenol 3's a day for other bodily pains?

The meaning of pain was also illustrated when, while visiting with Carlin at the local cafe, I winced in mirrored pain when he was telling me about some of his former injuries. I pointed this out to him, and noted that his pain memories could be vicariously experienced by someone (me) who had never sustained that particular type of injury. On the other hand, I have felt other pains, so I have a history of knowing what pain feels like generally. The activity of my norepinephrine system likely also engaged, giving me full attention to those pain memories.

Interestingly, like Glenn, Carlin reported feeling no pain when he self-inflicted cuts to his forearm, which I could relate to from my own era of self-harm. Reise has knifed himself in the abdomen; Ulmer's upper arms are covered in parallel, slashed scars from his prison days. Glenn's forearms are criss-crossed with jagged white lines. In all these cases, the meaning of the pain (anterior insula) was there without the (full) feeling of it (posterior insula). Indeed, research has shown that the insula is able to separate the emotional response to pain from the pain itself.[27]

Miguel has reported consistently that, in his experience, the street drug crystal methamphetamine

------

[27] Berthier 1988

can alter his experience of pain. Miguel, who suffers from severe arthritis and intense episodic bodily pains that come and go without warning, uses "dope" (crystal meth) to deal with his pain. "It doesn't take the pain away," he told me. "It takes away the focus on the pain. The pain is there but it's not registering." We at ACT, given that we are a mental health and addictions team operating under a provincial health authority, support our clients in decreasing or stopping drug use, but we also operate from a harm-reduction stance. With Miguel, when he tells me that his pain is "beyond 10/10" and that this is so unbearable that he uncharacteristically speaks of wanting to "jump in front of a bus" I take a harm-reduction stance: "Miguel, I'd rather see you use dope than kill yourself." The pain is still there when Miguel uses dope; it is still 10/10. It has simply lost its relevance. But when the pain strikes when he cannot use crystal meth, such as when he meets me at the ACT office and we go to a local coffee shop to visit, he writhes in unbearable pain. Often, the pain is his hand and travels: elbow, arm, spine; other times, his eyes water profusely as he rubs them and swears.

It sounds like his anterior and posterior insula are communicating differently when Miguel uses his drug of choice - if these areas are communicating at all then. Is Miguel's anterior insula put off-line by the meth, changing the meaning of Miguel's physical pain? Is the back of the insula still getting the information that pain in the body is present - signals from the pain receptors - but simply not passing this information on to the insular front lines? In other words, it sounds just like Miguel's description: the pain is there (in the posterior insula) but the meaning and focus of it all (anterior insula) doesn't register. It has been suggested that both pain and addiction involve the insula.[28] However, I could find nothing in the literature to support Miguel's claim of "dope" as a pain reliever/distractor, nor any studies to support - or, for that matter, refute - my hypothesis that meth interferes with the communication between the posterior and anterior regions of the insula. All I do know is that if Miguel finds relief in meth (he has been consistently unsuccessful in finding relief from other, conventional, pharmaceuticals) it just might save his life, and for that I am grateful.

Note, though, that as I write this, the "opioid epidemic" is in full force, and fentanyl is showing up in drugs other than opioids, including crystal meth. Miguel, and other users of meth, are at risk of overdosing on fentanyl any time they use. We at ACT, as well as many other sites in Vancouver, stress safer-using steps: Don't use alone. Try a test dose first. Carry Narcan/naloxone and know how to use it. Call 911 if a friend overdoses, even if they "wake up" from the Narcan and seem okay. I remind Miguel of this, concerned. It is complicated.

As we have seen, the salience of pain (self-inflicted, psychological, physical, etc.) can differ greatly from attention to that pain. Interestingly, norepinephrine can bias the formation of (pain?) memories towards being more salient than they otherwise would be.[29] Of note is glutamate's ability to

---

[28] Naqvi and Bechara 2009
[29] Mather et al. 2016

enhance norepinephrine's effects, and vice-versa,[30] thus implicating glutamate in salience again.

The salience network is thought to be highly disturbed, perhaps fundamentally, in schizophrenia (cause - or effect - of the VEN abnormalities, perhaps?). In fact, it has been proposed[31] that schizophrenia may be conceptualized as a disorder of the (mis)attribution of meaning, in which the illusion of meaning lurks behind the benign, and the meaningful stimuli of life are not assigned their proper significance. The network of salience has gone awry; we cannot choose by our own volition our own meanings.[32] I was prescient in my radio-interview definition of schizophrenia after all!

That salience network, finally

We constantly scan our environment and pick out what is meaningful to us; in other words, we notice what is *salient*. For example, when we look across a crowd to locate our friend, we do not have to focus on every single face; our brain (insula?) goes to work for us, and her face jumps out at us automatically and effortlessly. After all, our friend is salient to us. Researchers are fond of using tests such as showing their participants a page full of "T's" with a single (or a couple, depending on the study) odd-man-out "L's". The "L's" are difficult to locate unless they are, say, coloured pink in a sea of green "T's" in which case they seem to jump out at us, just

---

[30] ibid.

[31] e.g., Humpston 2017

[32] Hawkes 2012

like our friend's face in the crowd. In psychosis, abnormalities of salience are stopping at many faces and attributing a friend-like relationship to them, or not recognizing your friend at all. In other words, the insula and related areas may see meaning when there is none, or miss meaning that is there. I, for example, pick up garbage when I'm not well, thinking it holds momentous meaning for my life. Find a bullet-shaped piece of wood? I'm going to be executed by a sniper. A length of yellow plastic? My death will create a crime scene, with that yellow tape police use to communicate "Do Not Enter." To me, when I'm caught up in that meaning, it seems to be the most logical conclusion possible. On the other hand, I might feel no emotional reaction to a photo of a friend - I'm missing the meaning.

The anterior insula gets its information regarding meaning from both the external (e.g., auditory or visual stimuli) and the internal sensory systems (e.g., our sense of our internal states, whether cognitive, emotional, or visceral). Neurons in the anterior insula bring these two together in a meaning-making way, trying to achieve and maintain homeostasis. For most people, "I am hearing someone talking" and "I sense that what I am hearing is important to me" are experiences restricted to actual external voices and indices of personal significance. It is a reality-based (insular?) function, sewing our experiences into a coherent and meaningful tapestry. In contrast, schizophrenia hijacks the insula, artificially - but very convincingly - giving it the signal that the auditory part of the brain has heard something, and that it is personally relevant. This leaves the person with schizophrenia with the insular output of "that voice I just heard - I *know* in my gut, in my heart, that they are talking to me and have a message of importance and relevance." It brings together the external ("hearing") and the internal (visceral sensations "in my gut... in my heart") and leads us to perseverate in the delusions thus spawned.

Detection of reality is made even more difficult. The salience detection extends to the brain "hearing" its own noise and "feeling" its own gut even when these do not represent any actual inputs from the outside. When Carlin feels validity in his gut (via oxytocin?), in his core being, and the auditory trace in his brain is identical to that induced by physical sound waves, how can he not be compelled to believe? Carlin is "making meaning" in his salience network, trying to find the most plausible explanations possible. This perturbed sense of meaning has the potential to completely derail our mental health. It is the foundation of a psychotic disorder, in which we are disconnected - "broken off" - from reality. This explains the etymology of the term schizophrenia: "schizo" means "break" (i.e., "schism") and "phrenia" means "mind". This gives us a mind cut off from reality. Our broken salience networks are messing with our minds.

DMN it!

Another important task our salience network does is that it acts as a switch between two other network states. The first is our brains' "idling" mode, thanks to a network of neurons referred tongue-in-cheek to as the DMN: the *default mode network*. This DMN (consisting of the back region, or posterior, of the cingulate cortex (PCC) and the medial PFC) flickers on when we've finished a task and have yet to start the next, a kind of neural daydreaming. Your thoughts wander as you engage in some self-reflection, mental imagery, inner speech, and planning. Memory is reviewed, future plans appear, and emotions flit by. Normally, it is loose but coordinated. In schizophrenia, the DMN is poorly connected; multiple brain regions that are normally in sync show disturbed integration. Our autobiographical self that normally hums along with the DMN is disturbed in schizophrenia[33] and it is harder to monitor the self, particularly when adaptively changing from external to internal perspectives, and back again.

I am a DMN good brain wanderer. My thoughts (*that car's license plate has my initials, huh*) and emotions (free-range anxiety) lead my inner voice to create a dream-like story; only, I have schizophrenia, and these waking "dreams" quickly become nightmares. *The car with the EE license plate has stopped at the lights ahead... waiting for me to walk across... I'm sure he has a gun... if I look at him, he will shoot... if I ignore his power and don't look, he'll shoot... shit, I'm doomed.* All of a sudden it is no more a DMN humming along; I've exited into a harsh reality and I am on full alert. DMN it, I've lost sight of reality and am in imagined situations. My clients can identify.

The other main network influenced by the

---

[33] Berna et al. 2016

salience network is the CEN: the *central executive network*. It employs another part of the PFC (dorsolateral PFC or dlPFC) than the DMN does (medial PFC or mPFC). The main purpose of the CEN is the control of our higher cognitive functioning; none of this wishy-washy DMN activity. What we think, feel, and do is all affected by our CEN. It employs our working memory, a task the DMN cares very little about. The anterior insula, as part of our salience network, is key for the switching between the DMN and the CEN in a healthy way.

In schizophrenia, when the salience network is impaired, we may perseverate in behaviours that our CEN would normally tell us to let go of. Maybe the DMN gets too much say in these matters. Overall, in those with schizophrenia, there is unusual and inappropriate switching happening,[34] in response to salient events.[35] I notice a benign example of this often, when riding the bus and ear-budded into my iPod. A song I like comes up, and my DMN recedes as I realize, *Hey, I like this song. I want to pay attention so I don't miss my favourite part.* That attention lasts a moment or two, and, before I know it, the song has passed and I've missed that favourite part. My CEN, which I initially engaged to pay attention, has fallen to DMN mind wandering. Thanks to my salience network, I switched from DMN to CEN to DMN to CEN again. My DMN is inactive during the cognitively demanding task of attention, and my CEN goes off-line when my dreamy DMN takes over. In

---

[34] White et al. 2010
[35] Ham et al. 2013

this example, the failure to maintain CEN interest is mundane. But when schizophrenia takes over, the results can be difficult to live with. A prime example of this is the case of auditory hallucinations, a cardinal feature of schizophrenia that has been found to emerge from a dysfunctional insula operating within a disturbed salience network.[36]

---

[36] Palaniyappan and Little et al. 2012; Palaniyappan et al. 2011

Chapter 3

+When the Voices are Outside

They, the researchers, say it's our thoughts, megaphoned into existence by missing neurons and faulty wiring. This may well be true, but we who hear Voices (I think they deserve an uppercase "V" given their identities, volume, and variety) hear them vividly, coming to us as if from outside of us; as if sound waves were actually bending hairs in our cochleas and sending signals to our brains. That's what it sounds like, certainly. While some Voices are quieter, many are as loud as any human conversant, and we can even pinpoint the direction from which they are coming (mine tend to come from a few feet behind me, from over my right shoulder). To us, they are not "auditory verbal hallucinations" (AVHs) that our brains construct, but capital-V Voices. And, more often than not, they confuse us, hurt us, deceive us, direct us. We suffer.

Hearing Voices, and, especially, responding to them out loud, is in our society the epitome of "losing your mind" or being "schizo," "nuts," or, the ever popular "cra-a-zy" (finger twirling at the side of the head). It violates societal norms and engenders fear, not trust, by others. Soon, inputs of strange looks and avoidance behaviours give the person responding to his or her Voices aloud the feedback that others are not benevolent and cannot be trusted. There is the palpable feeling of being watched and judged. Given this culture of fear and mistrust, I had begun my visits with Carlin in true peer support fashion, relating how I myself know the experience of Voices. I think this gave Carlin a place of safety in which he might talk about his own. He began to talk freely, feeling unjudged and unhurried. I ask Carlin about his Voices every week, and we discuss them at length. Even on our visit the week of his birthday, when ACT traditionally treats the celebrant to a meal instead of just a coffee, he chose our usual Tim Horton's and launched into stories of his Voices right away.

"I'm glad I can talk to you about my Voices," Carlin stated that day. "I can't tell my Mom, people will think I'm crazy. Am I crazy?"

I smiled. "Only if I'm crazy too. You know about my Voices," I countered. Carlin smiled also, feeling heard, validated, and respected. He knew about my Voices.

Early on in our peer relationship, Carlin told me that he hears a recurring Voice, the Voice of a man saying, repeatedly, with an ominous tone, "Fuck you, fuck you, fuck you." Carlin has a clear sense that the man is holding a microphone, and he mimes the action each time he imitates this Voice. It is a calculated Voice, and a deep bass, which Carlin also mimics. He has told me about this Voice many times, and it clearly disturbs him. Of course it would disturb - the language is coarse and intent to harm clear; it is linked to Carlin's history of being beaten into a coma in his youth. This violent assault is what tore from Carlin the ability to walk and talk, ripping from him his dreams of playing professional sports. Carlin has learned, hard-fought, to manage his daily life, but certainly feels that, as the Voice says, he has been unfairly "fucked."

Other Voices talk about what Carlin is doing, or what he should/shouldn't be doing. Where I hear "she," Carlin hears masculine pronouns: "He's crossing the street." "He's finished his doughnut." They comment on what we are doing, mundanely, and then judge us. I notice mine are especially assaultive when I am, with my thoughts, berating myself; I must ask Carlin if he finds that too. He wondered aloud one week about their links to his inner world. Regardless, a near-constant prattle is what Carlin lives with. Occasionally, he tells me that they are "quiet" during our visits. Why? "They are listening… to get information," Carlin proposes. Their near-ubiquity means their absence, too, is relevant and in need of explanation. The silence is loud, we agreed.

Carlin is my client who keeps me most on my neuroscientific toes. Intelligent and perceptive, Carlin showed great interest when I talked about the brain and my Voices. At first, I explained things simplistically:

"You know how the brain's 'hearing area' is active when we hear a sound? Well, in some people and at some times, that area is active without any actual sound coming in."

Carlin nodded. This was the easy part. The next would be more vague, less precisely related to the science of Voice hearing. But I was looking to explain things simply; I know all too well the glazed-eye response when I wax too technical with clients (or my friends, for that matter; but they know I'm a nerd already and love me despite, or for, it). For Carlin, I had presented the peer support sentiments of understanding and non-judgment first, and, later, to fill in the neuroscientific gaps.

"Well, there's also an area on the brain that says, 'This Voice is coming from outside of me.' Anytime we hear someone say something to us, this area 'lights up.' What happens when we hear our Voices is that this area, along with that area of 'I am hearing a Voice' get active all on their own - without there actually being any actual Voice. The effect is this: we hear a clear Voice, and are given the message of 'outside of me.'"

I hadn't lost him. Carlin was nodding, and I remained firm in my belief of his intelligence. This would go on to be but one of our many talks about our brains. At one point, he started asking, "What's the neuroscience behind that?" He was gaining valuable insight into the symptoms of his schizophrenia, though of course I couldn't rationalize it all away for him. He remained fixed in his delusions, but was becoming open to explaining his hallucinations with neuroscience.

The neuroscience of Voices

Explaining auditory verbal hallucinations

(AVHs) with neuroscience would be a fairly straight-forward task, I assumed, when I began to research the topic for this chapter. Not so. Soon my own brain was swimming with: "neural oscillations... neural synchrony... gamma activity... corollary discharge..." and other brain-twisters. Nonetheless, let me try to capture it for you.

First, some neuroanatomy. The *primary auditory cortex* ("primary" meaning the "first" area that begins the process of identifying a sound) is located in the temporal lobes, hidden within the lateral sulcus (the gyrus involved is known as Heschl's gyrus): that is, a smallish area in each of the brain's hemispheres, buried right behind your ears. Strangely, sounds entering your left ear mostly end up in the right cortex and vice versa, after making a few pit stops (e.g., inferior colliculus, thalamus) along the way. (This is not much more intuitive than the visual system, in which the messages from your retinas reach all the way to the primary cortex in the occipital lobe, at the very back of your brain: we actually do have "eyes in the back of our heads"! But I digress.) This primary auditory cortex receives the electrochemical messages that each cochlea (in our inner ear) has concocted out of the physical stimuli of sound waves.

While we have these two spots of the brain responding to sound, one in each of the brain's hemispheres, they are not created equal, and for good reason. Think about it: the most common auditory input we humans know is speech. Brain regions like to specialize, to a certain extent, and language is a prime example. We have dedicated areas in the left temporal lobe for the comprehension of language (Wernicke's area), with the production of speech relying on a region in the left frontal lobe (Broca's area). (A minority of people, particularly those who are left-handed, have their speech centres in their right hemisphere, or divided left-right with more equality.) Although some people with schizophrenia hear non-speech hallucinations, such as that of the phone ringing or a train passing (which Glenn hears), 60-80% of people with schizophrenia hear verbal auditory hallucinations, or Voices. Carlin, Ulmer, Reise, and I all fall into that group.

But what's going on in our right primary auditory cortex? It has been proposed that the right hemisphere is about the emotional tones of the Voices, and the prosody or "music" of our speech. Would it have anything to do with the fact that most Voices are firmly derogatory in nature? "Stupid girl!" I hear. Words that are highly emotionally charged, such as curse words, may be associated with activity in the right temporal lobe. (Which explains how some elderly people, after a stroke affecting their left language centres, swear profusely despite living their whole lives before the injury as people who would not even "take the Lord's name in vain." They are simply trying to communicate with what they have, brain-wise, which is an intact right side.) It would make sense that Voices would be linked to the left; the right is likely where my musical hallucinations originate, and perhaps part of Carlin's "fuck you" Voice.

That the primary auditory cortex is disturbed in schizophrenia is evidenced by a reduction in its grey matter.[37] This loss correlates with Voice severity[38] - the more you've lost, the worse the Voices. In people at high risk for developing schizophrenia - those who have close relatives with schizophrenia, for example - there is also a loss of grey matter here, and the smaller the area of speech comprehension (the posterior superior temporal gyrus), the more likely it is that the high-risk person will go on to have full-on Voices. Grey matter loss means fewer neurons and less connectivity, a perfect storm for symptoms of mental illness.

So, since we know that the posterior superior temporal gyrus is connected to Voice-hearing, some researchers decided to try to "zap" them away, using a technique called TMS: transcranial (through the skull) magnetic (yes, magnets) stimulation (the "zap"). I've had this done to me, as part of a research study (though not to the auditory cortex for Voices, unfortunately), and I can attest to its painlessness. They simply place a magnetic coil on your skull and send in a magnetic current. Zap! It stuns the cortex into silence, even for many of the 25% of Voice-hearers whose Voices do not go away with antipsychotic medications - and the Voices are then absent for up to several weeks after a session! "Significant and large effects" were reported by one recent meta-analysis.[39] So cool, I thought, but was then disappointed that this procedure, despite becoming standard in some research circles, is not yet

---

[37] Mulert et al. 2011

[38] ibid.

[39] Freitas et al. 2009

standard in treatment regimes. I wish Carlin could try it, to see if the Voices he hears (that are indeed resistant to his hefty dose of medication; Carlin is among that unlucky 25%) could be affected by TMS. Its effects are specific to auditory hallucinations, not to schizophrenia more broadly. But it's certainly a good start, as Voices are arguably the most common, and cardinal, symptom of schizophrenia. And this can be devastating.

39 years of Voices

Ulmer ("the god of winter") hears the voices of the Christian God, Christ, Devil, and a variety of spirits, angels, and demons - as well as certain Hollywood celebrities and presumed family members. Sadly, he has been plagued by these Voices for decades - 39 years, to be exact; my age, we note. Ulmer and I bonded over coffee and stories of our Voices when I began working with him on ACT about four years ago.

Ulmer was intrigued by my experiences of Voice-hearing, and I was eager to share according to my new position as a peer support worker. This began in the local Starbucks. "You hear Voices?" he boomed. In a very loud voice, to make myself heard to his hard-of-hearing, I replied. Honestly. Soon, all the patrons in that Starbucks knew my experiences of hearing Voices. I was a bit embarrassed, speaking up so loudly, but he could not otherwise hear me. It built rapport with Ulmer, which is the basis of our peer relationship. Our subsequent visits over the past few years have made talking about our respective Voices an easy conversation. It often followed that the conversation went like this:

"I heard the Devil talking last night," he once began on one of our weekly visits. "He told me that he took my soul, but then God brought me back." His Voices often carried such religious themes. "My voices were bad then. All night. I said that she would intervene for me. Could you phone her and tell her that I'm waiting for her to come? She will come see me in 2018 [it was 2016 at the time], and she is my wife." His notation of "Voices" as such meant what he heard, nothing more, nothing less. They might be more or less bothersome, but never unreal. He was certain of this, and emphatic.

"You guys just call it delusional, all in my head. You don't believe me."

True. His Voices say things that are clearly not based in reality. I believed in his suffering, though - just not in its basis. Could that be enough for peer support? Was there a way to acknowledge that pain without saying that what he hears is indeed "all in his head" (that is, all in his brain)? His insula may have been helping to make the auditory hallucinations he hears and his "gut" intuitions he has into a coherent story ("She's coming to see me in 2018."). Perhaps, when he hears Isabella's Voice, he is moved so deeply that it would be sacrilege to discount it as not-real. It is prominent, very notable, to Ulmer. His salience network - recall that circuit of neurons that prompt us about what to focus our attention and resources on - must be in overdrive.

In the end, I gave Ulmer an addressed and stamped envelope to his "famous wife, Isabella" - that is, addressed to her fan club. I judiciously did not tell him this last bit. It is now in his hands to write to her, and I hope that this will reduce or even eliminate Ulmer's constant asking for us at ACT to contact her and "tell her I'm waiting." The lines are so blurred and grey: what is supporting the emotional content of a person's deeply held beliefs and what is feeding a delusion? Is making him feel heard and respected outweighing the negativity of a false pretense? God help me... just don't let "Him" speak to me![40]

Waves, and lighting up

When most people think of research and the study of the brain, they think of pictures, with coloured parts of the brain "lighting up" (note: the researchers add the "lit" colours; they simply code for the activity levels). These images show us where things are happening. While these have their place, a different method for studying the brain is of note here. The EEG (electroencephalogram) measures the electrical currents of the brain, since the activity of firing an action potential is a form of electricity, a movement of ions. When large groups of neurons fire together in synchrony, the signal can be picked up by electrodes placed just on the subject's scalp. Since electricity is a quick phenomenon - here and gone in an instant - we can say *when* the activity is happening, on the scale of milliseconds (i.e., the *temporal resolution* of the EEG is good). However, recording from the scalp means not being as sure of *where* that activity is

---

[40] Sadly, in the time between writing this manuscript and its final editing, Ulmer died of a drug overdose. Given the Covid-19 pandemic at the time, we could not even gather for a memorial for Ulmer.

coming from (i.e., EEGs have poor *spatial resolution*). Compare this with the "picture" MRI or CT scans: these methods are good at the *where* but less so on the *when*.

I've had the pleasure of participating in some EEG research studies. They put a cap of many electrodes (256, in my experience, though sometimes as few as four are used) on my head, with a few electrodes on my face. A soapy saline solution is used to help the current pass from scalp to electrode, which tickles as the researcher squirts it on each lead. That is the extent to which you feel anything; the EEG itself is painless. The electrodes are recording, not zapping. It can last for anywhere between a few minutes to half an hour or more. Just like in the movies, the electrical signals - "brain waves" - are scratched out by fine pens onto a rolling paper or similarly recorded by a connected computer. You can get a lot of data, really fast, and fairly cheaply.

EEGs are best known for their use in medical investigation and research on epilepsy. If someone has a suspected seizure disorder, they will undergo an EEG. A seizure looks like a spasm of activity in the EEG readout: tall waves, close together. This offers the diagnosis of epilepsy, and can give the physician a general idea of where the seizure's focus is, but not a precise location. In other words, it tells them where to check more closely with another technique.

A normal EEG reveals the variety of brain waves we have, and these are classified according to their frequency (in Hertz, Hz, which means oscillations per second): the back-and-forth of firing/resting from action potentials. At the moment, I hope you are experiencing lots of beta "busy" waves (16-31 Hz): that you are alert, focused, and actively thinking... though too much of a good thing means that your beta waves may be also associated with anxiety. Then, you need a "beta break," a return to the alpha waves (8-15 Hz) that are correlated with relaxation and reflection. Later, when you are drowsy and ready for bed (maybe you are reading this under the covers?), you will likely be idling, with theta waves (4-7 Hz); once you've slipped into a good sleep, your brain will be dominated by the slow delta (< 4 Hz) waves.

Then there are the high-frequency gamma waves (40-100 Hz), the state of a brain "in sync." Think of an orchestra as it warms up - musical chaos. Then, in comes the conductor, and at his commands, they play beautifully, in synchrony. Gamma waves are that coherent coming together of different neural "sounds" and are the opportunity of a lifetime for the learning brain. As more and more brain areas "fire together," their neurons "wire together": the brain reprograms, balances, problem-solves. Ah ha! Sudden insights appear and intuitive solutions burst out spontaneously with those gamma waves. You are by no means on autopilot anymore; you are profound and think of new ways of doing things. Beta waves might have gotten you part-way there, but they are a bit too chaotic; gamma activity brings you into clear focus. Signals from your emotional brain are quieted. It is not surprising that the brains of experts in meditation are brimming with gamma waves.[41]

---

[41] Kingsland 2016

This made me so excited, thinking of my own brain's potential for gamma activity. Surely I had deep insights and problem-solving going on - I'm writing a book on the neuroscience of schizophrenia, after all. Schizophrenia. Right. The disease I have, and one, I now know, that is associated with reduced gamma activity. We could be considered as being stuck in beta, not progressing to the wonderful gamma activity. What, I then wondered, about the almost excess of "ah ha!" moments and the bringing together of different bits of information for the formation of complex theories? We who suffer from schizophrenia experience insights to the nth degree, at times too much connection. Sure, they are delusional, paranoid, and based on hallucinations, but does that condemn us to live in beta? Maybe we are more in need of meditations, not just medications.

Back to the Voices

Let's return to the topic of this chapter now, that of Voices (as I've stated, physicians and researchers call them auditory verbal hallucinations, or AVHs, but I will continue to call them Voices, as it reminds us of the quality of Voice-ness reality they come with). There is a reason we took that electroencephalographic detour: the notion that we need to "synch before you speak."[42] In one study,[43] the participants alternated between saying "ah" and hearing "ah." In the healthy controls, there was a moment of synchrony right before they spoke - but

[42] Ford et al. 2007
[43] see Uhlhaas et al. 2008 for a review

not when they listened. It was as if the command to speak also sent a synchronizing message to the sensory cortex: *I am about to move my lips and tongue to say something. So if you sense something in those places, don't worry - it's just me.* But in the participants who had schizophrenia - those who experienced Voices - there was markedly less synchrony, with the severity of the Voices correlating with a more chaotic, less "in sync" brain.

Does this mean the people with Voices were not getting that crucial message (*don't worry, it's me speaking*) as they said the "ah"? The experience of Voices are thus seen as an equivalence between "I thought that" and "I heard that." We don't record them as their own thoughts, memories, or other inner experiences; they are perceived as someone else's words. External words. Out loud. Voices.

This is known as the corollary discharge hypothesis, and involves the motor areas in the frontal lobe telling the primary auditory cortex (we know it's Heschl's gyrus, to be precise) in the temporal lobe the message to *be prepared!* for the upcoming speech. In hearing Voices, this area is likely active without the usual restraints: in Carlin, his primary auditory cortex may often be up and running before any external sound activates it. According to the corollary discharge hypothesis, it is his inner linguistic thoughts that are prodding the temporal lobe - but without the tag that they are exactly that: his. *Oh,* Carlin's auditory centres say. *I haven't received news from the frontal motor areas that we are moving our lips and tongue for speech. This mustn't be ours. I must be "hearing things."* This is related to the finding that the auditory N100 (a normal, negative EEG spike in response to hearing something; it occurs about 100 milliseconds after the onset of the auditory stimulus) is not suppressed in schizophrenia when we speak; this contrasts to the norm (i.e., in people without schizophrenia), in which the N100 is suppressed when speech is self-generated.[44]

That suppression is generally associated with a *synchrony of oscillations* that an EEG picks up. Think of a room of grandfather clocks, each with their own oscillating pendulums. Each clock represents a smaller group of neurons that are in sync, whose activity swings back and forth, actively firing axon potentials and resting, and active again. Then try to get all the clocks to swing (oscillate) together, until you get the whole room in beautiful synchrony. Not so easy. But our brains manage quite well, in their circuits. So that's what the EEG picks up: a roomful of grandfather clocks. Remember the brain wave frequencies? They represent the coordinated oscillations of millions of neurons in the brain (and the frequency of their oscillations correspond to the alpha, beta, theta, delta, and gamma waves observed). The strength of the synchrony predicts correct responses in lab animal study settings,[45] but my or Carlin's brain would have difficulties in (humanly) equivalent lab tasks. This makes sense: my or Carlin's "brain of grandfather clocks" would have a lot of confusing noise, if our schizophrenia is making us have trouble synchronizing.

---

[44] Heinks-Maldonado et al. 2007

[45] Kreiter and Singer 1996

So the neurons of the primary auditory cortex are acting strangely. Moreover, researchers have found that there are actually fewer neurons there to begin with in those with schizophrenia, that grey-matter volume deficit. Specifically, one meta-analysis - in which data from over 300 Voice-hearing people with schizophrenia were examined - found that there were reductions in the grey matter volume of that temporal lobe.[46] Is Carlin coping with fewer neurons in this area? Is that what's keeping him from getting that corollary discharge? Is no one around in his auditory centres to receive the messages of "this is me"?

Were Carlin's or my brain being studied while we hear our Voices, there would likely be "abnormal function." The theory is simple: fewer grey-matter neurons means less connectivity; less connectivity may mean Carlin's brain can't block the normal attribution of inner speech, memories, and experiences as inner. Some inhibition is lacking; some GABA interneurons aren't there to inhibit crucial circuits. Structural/connectivity problems are nothing new to schizophrenia researchers, who have found these problems in many brains, by many methods. Schizophrenia is believed to be a developmentally-based disorder of brain structures, and, by extension, connectivity. The grey matter that is lost is in the areas in which neurons make their synaptic connections, so it makes sense that impaired connectivity is correlated with structural abnormalities. Which came first, disruption of

---

[46] Modinos et al. 2012

structure or of function, is as difficult to determine as the chicken and the egg dilemma.

Interestingly, the last time I spoke with Carlin, he recounted to me a detailed and vivid "memory" of his birth. "I was in red, when suddenly I was being squeezed through a... place," he said delicately. "Then everything was bright and loud, and I think I was crying." I'll leave aside the contentious nature of our being able to remember anything before about three years of age (and birth memories are particularly untenable, according to memory researchers), when our hippocampi - bilateral subcortical structures crucial for memory - mature. Instead, Carlin's story reminded me that birth traumas and complications are associated with schizophrenia,[47] although it may also be that there are neurodevelopmental problems in the brains of people who later develop schizophrenia, and these may be happening in the brain even before birth. That developmental problem may be related to the lack of synchrony found in the brains of people who live with schizophrenia. Synchrony drives specific connectivity,[48] and ordered oscillations drive the developmental- and learning-based pruning of synapses.[49] Is there a vicious cycle at work: less synchrony meaning abnormally-pruned groups of neurons, which then leads to insufficient synchrony? Does schizophrenia get us coming and going?

Similarly, schizophrenia gets us front-and-back

---

[47] Cannon et al. 2002

[48] Uhlhaas et al. 2010

[49] Uhlhaas et al. 2008

with gamma activity. Earlier, we noted that there is, as a general rule, less gamma activity in the brains of people living with schizophrenia. But it turns out that there is an interesting exception to this rule: in the left primary auditory cortex of people who experience Voices there is an increase of gamma activity.[50] So we have too little gamma activity when and where we need it and too much of it when and where we don't. In those of us with schizophrenia, our cortical auditory areas go hyper-excitable with gamma activity, which suggests an obvious way to make Voices. Support for this idea also comes from the fact that TMS, which reduces cortical excitability, temporarily stops Voices. Hmm... I'm wondering about how Carlin's Voices often recede during our visits. Is my quiet presence and our engaging conversation kicking Carlin's cortex to simmer down, be less "excitable"?

That still leaves us with the question of where the content of Voices comes from. I, and I would bet Carlin as well, would have objections to the notion that our Voices are simply our inner thoughts, bull-horned. They may be verbal, as our thoughts tend to be, but they are experienced as foreign to our ways of thinking: *Not me.* My Voices can swear and are extremely derogatory, a far cry from my own lack of profanity and animosity in my thoughts and words. To think that our Voices can only access the language centres of our brains seems simplistic. Why not access our memories, hopes, and beliefs? After all, our brains are so interconnected. Think of how

---

[50] Mulert et al. 2011

dreams are made: various, and at times remote, regions of our brains are spontaneously active, which our subconscious weaves into a semi-coherent dream that feels, for the moment, real. Could our Voices similarly be a manifestation of a lot of diverse, underlying brain activity? Could, for example, my Voices of "She's bad, she's done for!" take cues from my paranoia ("people talk about me when they think I can't hear them and refer to me as 'she'"), my memories (in high school, I remember having heard people talking behind my back), my innermost fears ("I'm not a worthwhile person"), and my dashed ("done for") hopes of being a PhD-holding neuroscientist with my own laboratory (a long-held dream schizophrenia took away from me). Could my foreign-feeling Voices be based on a weird combination of all these mental states? Perhaps when Ulmer tells me that his Voices say to him: "Your wife, Isabella, is coming to reunite with you in 2018!" they are his hopes for someone to change his life for the better: his loneliness; his memories of belonging to a family; his desire to be connected to something bigger than himself (Isabella and her fame).

So is there altogether a problem with incoming sensory stimuli, internally stored information, and outgoing messaging - and the brain's attempts to integrate them all? It would make sense that a lot of processes could be involved, even in just the experiences of Voices. There certainly are commonalities: that they are usually Voices (but not always; sometimes they are mechanical sounds); that these Voices are often derogatory; that they at most times are recognizable as human, and often as people we have known or wish to know; that they come from a definable place in space; and that they differ in volume and intensity. But just as each person - Voice-hearer or not - is unique, so also are those stimuli in our environments, the information we have stored in our brains, and the messages we are thinking about. We can study Voices as a category, but when I sit down with Carlin at the local Tim Horton's, I don't relate to him as a bundle of mixed messages in his brain meeting the bundle of mixed messages in my brain. I listen to the distress he is bearing, how it relates to his own history, and how he perceives both his present and his hopes for his future. I hope I help alleviate his suffering; indeed, he seems eager to talk to me most times I go knocking on his door. So, we talk about Voices.

Chapter 4

But I *Know* It: Delusions, Paranoia, and Memory of the Future

They're watching me.

Egocentric? Perhaps. But when your brain is off-kilter, you are utterly convinced of the surveillance, and it is terrifying. This schizophrenic paranoia can destroy your life. You can't trust anyone, and any of their attempts to intervene - for your own well-being - may provoke you to accuse them, push them away. The circle of impact grows.

It doesn't help matters that Vancouver boasts a shop called "The Spy Store." Or turn on your TV, and see reality stars under surveillance 24/7. Social media is ubiquitous. Ride the bus or enter a store: cameras; microphones. *This call will be recorded for quality assurance.* I cannot honestly tell my clients that they are not being watched. Unfortunately, the very existence of these technologies - such as tiny, miniature cameras and microphones - sometimes offers ideas that those of us prone to paranoia fall deeply into.

I have been in that place of paranoia. I feared for my life when my schizophrenic brain convinced me that a neighbour was bugging my apartment, tracking my movements, and had a sniper gun pointed at me waiting for the right time to kill me. Terror reigned, and I did things that were definitely not normal in my attempts to keep myself safe, to find a place where surveillance was off and privacy was restored. It was emotionally exhausting.

Given that the majority of my clients, like me, have schizophrenia, it is not surprising that paranoia shows itself often (as in, "paranoid schizophrenia" though this term is used less often now than even 20 years ago when I was diagnosed). When paranoia does rear its scary head, the flavour of the fear is relatively the same from person to person - we are genuinely and deeply affected - while the content of the paranoia varies greatly. There are themes, though, and these change consistently from era to era, depending on the technologies and fears of the age. Decades ago, it was not uncommon for someone with schizophrenia to believe that they had a radio transistor in their tooth; that is, their beliefs were in line with the science and technology of their time. In these years, the 2010's-2020's, things are more complex. For example, when Carlin received his first hearing aids, they demonstrated the tiny microphones that made them work. He emerged from the exam room, exclaiming to his mother and me who were waiting for him, "It's the microphone! It's so tiny, it's how they put the one in my throat!" Carlin had long believed that there was some recording being done on him, and now technology had given him the plausibility of this implausible belief. In paranoia, the proof of possibility seems to cement any actuality.

"I know it."

I would assume that the paranoia that you are being followed has remained fairly consistent across the decades, and even centuries, as carefully shadowing someone is not by definition technology-dependent. Take Miguel's beliefs, for example. For quite some time now, Miguel has been adamant that he is being watched by the Vancouver Police Department (VPD): "I walk down an alley, and there they are. At the park. On the bus. Everywhere."

"How do you know that they're cops?" I ask, conveying curiosity instead of judgment.

"Oh, I *know*. They look just like cops. That girl on the bus here - she had a ponytail. She was a cop."

"Was she in uniform?"

"No," Miguel said. "But I could tell, how she dressed."

"It's possible that she just dressed that way. People do, right? And even if she was one, how do you know she was surveilling *you*?" I asked.

Again, the unwavering assertion: "Oh I *know*."

It always seems to come back to that feeling of *knowing*. When we have that gut-level certainty, we dismiss almost any evidence to the contrary. The problem is that that "feeling" is not trustworthy and can be the result of the misfiring of some specific neural circuits. Yet, even when it seems preposterous, many people with schizophrenia will go to great lengths to explain their *knowing*.

One of my clients *knows* that people are stealing from him; another *knows* that things are appearing out of nowhere in his apartment due to people planting them there. Both have told me many elaborate explanations in their attempts to explain their predicaments. The explanations fit on differing points along the continuum of the possible, the plausible, and the impossible. I try to sort out those points with them.

"I left the cigarettes right there, on the coffee table," Carlin said with conviction. "They're gone."

A reasonable thing to wonder about.

"In that wall, there, beside the table. That's where they made the hole. Then they reached in and took them." I saw no flaw in the wall, but then, Carlin informed me, they had closed it over again after the meddling. His mind knew that he had to explain why he could no longer see the hole, and while my mind went to the conclusion that there probably wasn't a hole, Carlin went to other great explanatory lengths.

"How did they get to your wall?" I asked, knowing that he was a couple of stories up. I was trying to be logical, as if science could override a delusion (it can't). Still, I wanted to provoke him to test his own ideas.

"They can do it. I just *know* it. They're messing with me."

"Okay, that's one explanation. Can you think of any other ways your cigarettes went missing?"

"No, the hole. They're using it to spy on me too." This Carlin also *knew*.

Later, another day, Carlin told me that they were now returning things to him via this presumed hole. I tried another approach. "How many steps does your explanation take, Carlin? First, this person had to find out where you live (Step 1), bring a ladder (Step 2), cut a hole (Step 3), take the pack of cigarettes (Step 4), cover the hole (Step 5), leave/come back/do it again (Steps 6, 7 and 8) and return them (Step 9). They would have to know when you'd be at home or out (Step 10) and where you had put the pack (Step 11).

"Can I offer another possibility? Just a possible explanation, not necessarily the right one. Here: accidentally misplace the pack (Step 1) then find them (Step 2)."

"But - !"

"Yes, I know you don't remember that, and I'm not saying that that's what happened. I'm just suggesting another possible explanation, in addition to yours."

"Okay...."

"So, there's this principle in science, and it might work here, it might not. It's called 'Ockham's Razor'" (Carlin smiled at this.) "and it means that the simplest explanation, the one with the fewest steps is usually the right one. Usually, not always. Another way of saying it is - have you heard the phrase? - 'If you hear hoof beats, think horses, not zebras.'"

"So you're saying...?"

"Just because an explanation is possible, even plausible, doesn't necessarily make it right. Here in Canada, if you hear hoofbeats, it's going to be a common horse, not an exotic zebra. You have to think of different scenarios, compare them, then decide for yourself. I'm not going to tell you how they could be stealing from you; I just want to say, it's probably not a 'zebra.' But in the end, it's your decision, and it will affect how you deal with the situation."

I spoke bluntly because I knew Carlin well, and knew he was often influenced by logical theorizing. I wanted him to know that I, someone he trusted, had my own take on the situation, meaning that he wasn't necessarily confined to his current explanations. In general with my clients, I try to offer alternates while emphasizing the fact that while something can be possible (after all, have you ever played the lotto?) plausibility should be considered in our judgments. Interestingly, months later, Carlin hasn't been mentioning the hole, despite the fact that his things are still going missing and being re-found. Perhaps he may be ready to look for horses now?

Listening to your gut, following your heart

Knowing that something is salient and at least possible may lead off in several different directions. One is the trailblazing, ahead-of-his-time pioneer; another connects with others who are similarly convinced, regardless of the veracity. Some, whose brains are vulnerable, veer off into paranoia. This is when the *knowing* haunts you, and you are suffering.

That feeling of *knowing* is, of course, based in neurobiology. But before tackling the brain's role in this, we move first to the gut and the heart. Remember how the brain has about 100 billion (100,000,000,000) neurons? Well, the gut has a surprising 100 million (100,000,000) neurons: the size of a cat's brain! True, most of them are concerned with digestion, but many send and receive messages to and from the brain in our skull. The heart, likewise, has neurons, though only about 40,000 of them. These two organs have been shown repeatedly to be able to influence brain activity via this connectivity. Reflecting this, we have many phrases in the English language that emphasize how we feel when we are utterly certain of something: *"I feel it in my gut." "Her story was heart-felt." "That was a gut-wrenching movie." "My heart of hearts says so."* Indeed, we feel physical sensations in the areas of our gut and heart, especially when we are contemplating something meaningful to us.

There is a nerve, the vagus ("wandering") nerve, one of the longest nerves in the human body, that meanders through our body's organs, with the goal of bringing information from such places as the gut and the heart to the brain. Luckily for us, our visceral organs can function very well without much - or any - conscious effort on our part. On the other hand, our brains can also send overrides to our other organs. For example, when you are hungry, your gut tells your brain to organize some behaviours that would procure you some food, but your brain can also tell your gut that it's not going to get to eat, such as when you are "on a diet" and don't want to eat at every gut-based cue. However, when our feeding and gut feeling match, it makes us feel good, so it shouldn't be all that surprising that 95% of our serotonin (a "feel good" neurotransmitter) is found in the gut.

Then there's the heart, in which oxytocin can be released.[51] We've seen oxytocin already, in Chapter

---

[51] Jankowski 1998, 2000

1, where we explored its role in trust and other forms of bonding. But here, in the heart, its release may be the reason we say something is *"heart-felt"*: we are being bathed in that oxytocin.

"That was heart-stopping!" we might exclaim after an emergency, and it reminds us that changes in our heartbeat is a very physical manifestation of our emotional state, one which responds to oxytocin. An "exciting" experiment[52] neatly showed how a level of physiological arousal (including heart rate) affects our brain's conclusions and can result in the misattribution of arousal. Involved in this study were a swinging suspension bridge, a solid bridge, an attractive female among the researchers, and a number of male participants. The men were under the impression that the study was about some other, non-arousing task, but they had to cross one of the two types of bridges to get to the (attractive, female) researcher. It is no stretch to see that the men who crossed the swing-bridge were more aroused, in terms of increased heart-rate, shortness of breath, and mental alertness. (My heart certainly reacted when I embarked on a small suspension bridge!) What was interesting was that the men who crossed the swaying bridge tended to attribute their arousal not to the bridge but to the female waiting for them at the other end (they measured this by her giving her phone number to the men, and then they counted the number of men in each condition that phoned her). So an increased heartbeat can make your brain say, "I'm aroused!" instead of the other way around. (Of note,

---

[52] Dutton and Aron 1974

they found that the men were unaware that they were making this conclusion.)

Another client, Reise, seeks the opposite of the excited, aroused state: he has found gentle, mindful yoga and resting comfortably on his bean bag chair to be excellent ways to de-stress (i.e., reduce arousal). Since the vagus nerve runs by our lungs, deep breathing exercises such as those used in yoga can be very calming (which is also why we emphasize deep breathing with Glenn when his anxiety appears). This vagus nerve then passes the gut and heart en route to the brain, collecting data: *Slow heart-beat, easy digestion... I must be calm,* says the subconscious. "I *know* that this is good for me," seems to be Reise's conscious response.

The perspective your heart and gut tell you is worth listening to. I wonder if these organs may receive intuitions first, before your conscious brain does. So, perhaps we really should *listen to our gut and follow our heart.* Maybe *knowing* has some valuable perspectives. At least, that's what every taker of a multiple-choice exam relies on at times: the first, intuitive answer is often the correct one. Unless, that is, you are prone to delusion and paranoia. Then, all bets are off.

I wished I could see it

Another client, Miguel, does not attribute his unusual findings to others' actions, instead *knowing* that what he finds in his apartment is coming from his own body. Many visits have begun with his accounts. "I've got more stuff coming out of me," he says, then elaborates. "I cleaned my bathtub" (or floor or bed);

99

"it was spotless. Then I find it, like glue gun glue, strings, feathers or metal filings... I was in the clean bath (or floor or bed). It came out of my face" (or foot or other parts of his body). Sometimes, he brings samples, though more often than not, he doesn't. I encourage video recording, to bring this bodily feat to life for others, the ones he's trying to convince: me, the physician he trusts at ACT, and other team members.

For a long time, I didn't know what to do with this. Then, one day, as we sat on our bench at a local park in summer, Miguel took off his shoe and sock to show me first-hand the oddity of his "stuff coming out of me." I peered at his bare foot as he scraped and squeezed with his fingernails. "See? See it? It's right there. Oh, it's a big one!" I looked closer, thankful that he bathes regularly and lotions his feet profusely. I saw marks that looked like he had scraped his foot too hard with his nails, but I saw no "thing" coming out. "Oh wow, look at that!" Miguel exclaimed. He reached over to the ground and picked up part of a dirty, old cigarette filter that had been on the ground since long before we'd sat down. "Look at that. That came out of me." But it hadn't.

"That was there before," I said, but Miguel didn't hear me. He was intent on the next "thing."

"Incredible. Look!" Miguel exclaimed. I peered at his toe, where he was pointing. I looked, closely, and really, really hard.

I was honest: "I don't see it."

"You can't see that?"

"No, I can't."

"What's wrong with your eyes?"

He began picking at a piece of dried glue on his bag, which was under his foot. It too had been there since before he had removed his socks and shoes, but Miguel claimed it to be the next "thing coming out of my body." Later, it was another piece of something from off the ground. It was a bizarre mixture of hallucination - he could clearly see these things as he picked them out - and delusion: he was expecting something, and so looked (on the ground) until he found something that fit his ideas and perceptions. When I commented on this, he said, "It just shoots out. It's liquid, then it solidifies. See?" He held the glue in the palm of his hand and let me see it again. What could I say?

I could offer the more obvious (to me) explanations, but he has heard those and *knows* that they are wrong. At this point, I offer the listening ear, a sounding board, where he can express his thoughts, his *knowing*. It doesn't matter to me what, exactly, is going on; the greater issue is Miguel having a place to voice what he *knows*. With regards to other improbable-but-possible conclusions he may jump to, Miguel sometimes accuses his "friends" of stealing certain items from him only for him to find them later in another place. Due to this tendency (I have heard it from Miguel a number of times) I do stress to him that he has often assumed theft when in fact that was an incorrect assumption. It might have seemed possible and even plausible, but this *knowing* led him to the wrong interpretation. *Delay judgment as long as possible* applies here. Interestingly, Miguel recently had his intramuscular injections of an antipsychotic reinstated after a period of being off it, and since then he has rarely told me about "stuff coming out of" his body, and even the bit he refers to has not been with his former emphasis. This is correlation at this point, but it could be the beginning of finding causality. It wouldn't be the first time antipsychotics influenced "gut" and "heart" *knowing*.

Co-incidents

How did Miguel get into such a state? Likely, his glutamate and GABA have been exciting and inhibiting particular neurons and networks, including the activity of the coincidence detectors (NMDA receptor activation). This means that he can detect co-incidents: events that occur at the same time, such as his scraping his feet and finding bits of things on the ground. I hyphenate the word "co-incident" to highlight that they are simply two events happening close together in time and space. I am not making any claims regarding the almost spiritual sense we have when things occur together despite having a high unlikelihood of this happening.

In the brains of people living with schizophrenia, our excess of dopamine (in the ventral tegmental area, or VTA) makes these co-incidents very salient. Salience grabs Miguel's attention and makes him want to search for an explanation. His amygdala hates uncertainty and does not tolerate ambiguity, so Miguel is prone, prompted by that dopamine, to make spurious associations. This calms his discomfort of not being able to explain something. In turn, these beliefs can influence his perceptions: Miguel truly believed things were coming out of him, so much so that they self-reinforced and he - but not I

- could actually see the supposedly embedded objects. It becomes a circle of cause and effect: we humans tend to see what we believe, and to believe what we see.

The challenges of challenge

Interestingly, there is an observed paradox in which the tenacious delusional convictions held by people with schizophrenia are actually strengthened by being challenged,[53] and I see this in Carlin. The learning and memory paradigm explains this by the fact that a challenge forces the person to bring their delusion to the forefront of their consciousness - for example, making Carlin's memory imprint of the microphones active yet again by inquiring how he has been feeling about them. It is Hebbian synaptic learning at its best: when the presynaptic neuron fires repeatedly onto an active postsynaptic neuron, you will eventually get the postsynaptic outcome even with just a fraction of the input originally required. A mention of hearing aids caused Carlin to leap to his delusions of tiny microphones; I don't have to prompt his memory with a detailed synopsis of microphones and their incompatibility with throats. However, there is hope. It may be that when I cause Carlin to engage with his delusions, a labile state may arise.[54] This is a therapeutic window in which I just might be able to destabilize the delusions. Do I have just the right timing, compassion, and insight? I must tread carefully here, as I am just as likely to be reinforcing

---

[53] Corlett et al. 2010
[54] ibid.

and making him re-remember the very delusions I want to disrupt. Most of all, I do not want to disrupt our peer relationship of trust and rapport by having this conversation at the wrong time.

Making meaning

The line between delusion and paranoia is not always clear. When Carlin's belief about the microphone is not based in reality (delusion) it can combine with the fear he feels about being monitored (paranoia); they come together to cause him true suffering. These errors, being encoded by Carlin's insula and other related areas in his brain, lead, as we have seen, to things becoming more salient and significant than they should be. His amygdala, that centre for emotional experience, allocates more emotional attention to these salient things. There is fear generated by this amygdala activation, as the amygdala is particularly fond of negative emotions, but it is in the wrong context and he can't shake off the feelings of paranoia.

We don't often step back from our pill-centred, pharmaceutically-driven era, and we forget how astounding it is that we have found medicines, those antipsychotics, that can neurochemically address delusion and paranoia. A mere chemical in a tiny tablet taken by mouth with a sip of water could change that complex, all-consuming *knowing* and resultant fear of being watched or interfered with? The biochemistry of antipsychotic drugs in our schizophrenic brains and the neurophysiology underlying our beliefs can interact, at times with life-changing results - I know this in part because I am living it. If only that were true for more of us; despite regular medication, Carlin continues to hear Voices tell him he is going to die very soon, and the related paranoia leaves him with fear. Carlin's intelligence has required him to develop a complete and complex explanation for these ideas and emotions that his schizophrenia summons. He has to have it all make sense, to tie it all together. The problem is, as we discussed in the last chapter, he is being given false information by his Voices and his schizophrenia's excess of dopamine may be making it unnaturally hyper-salient. It is very, very hard for someone with schizophrenia to change their beliefs, no matter how "wrong" they are, because these beliefs make their experiences understandable and unified, instead of senseless and disjointed.

That (doesn't) remind me of...

We could also think of delusional beliefs as typical learning and memory gone awry. They explain the past and predict the future; yes, memory is not only concerned with retrieving the past, but also lets us create and evaluate scenarios that could be in our future. This "memory of the future"[55] lets us conceptualize possibility and probability, and guides our behaviour. It involves using cognition to evaluate possible strategies and emotions to guide intuitively, while also accessing memories for help when deciding on the best course of action - in light of past events. This all can be as detailed as any "normal" memory of the past. For example, consider this

---

[55] Szpinar et al. 2013

research paradigm:[56] participants were asked to imagine a future camping trip and the tools that would be needed; then, to remember a past camping trip (tools too); and, a hypothetical camping trip's tools. The participants' responses (number of tools remembered) varied according to how personally relevant the scenarios were, not how they fit in a past/future dichotomy. You can plan for the future based on recall of what you have experienced in the past. Just like you can remember familiar things more easily than unfamiliar ones, so also planning for the future is easier when the elements (particularly people) are familiar. Likewise, we remember and predict with more detail when the subject matter is familiar. Positive ones "stick" better than negative ones.

We are constantly evaluating how what we've learned matches up with our expectations, utilizing both our memory of both the past and of the future. When this fails - when what you expected to happen doesn't happen - it is termed a *prediction error*, and is particularly common in people with schizophrenia. Likely this is due to our having too much dopamine around. Normally, when a prediction error occurs, we go back and correct our assumptions, but when you have schizophrenia, it is as if you over-learn the first salient co-incidence, regardless of its veracity. Think of Miguel and his "things coming out": he doesn't look for further explanatory cues. Instead, the first-learned association is recalled and believed. As with any memory, each time you dredge it up, for

---

[56] ibid.

better or for worse you reinforce it. Add to that a PFC that isn't properly controlling your habenula (a tiny nucleus of neurons involved in reward prediction) and your commitment to your learned (though false) memories becomes highly tenacious. People with schizophrenia are more susceptible than the average person to thinking that an untrue memory they hold, even a benign one unrelated to their psychosis, is necessarily true (a memory illusion).[57]

The brain area most concerned with learning and memory, as we've hinted in previous chapters, is the hippocampus. This seahorse-shaped area ("hippocampus" comes from the Greek word for "seahorse") sits under the cortex of the temporal lobe and connects to a variety of regions we've discussed, including the amygdala (thanks to which the emotional tones of our memories are particularly vivid) and the PFC. The neuroscience of the hippocampus is complex and detailed, and I will not delve into it here. Suffice it to say that there are countless articles available online regarding its neuroanatomy, biochemistry, and connectivity, if you're interested. Here, our greatest concern is how the hippocampus relates to schizophrenia more generally.

Structurally, for those of us who live with schizophrenia, the hippocampus is smaller than average, by about 4%.[58] This sounds rather insignificant, but is actually a very robust and important finding. It is the most consistent structural

---

[57] Corlett et al. 2010
[58] Nelson et al. 1998 in Heckers 2001

abnormality found in schizophrenia. It was discovered more than 30 years ago[59] and has been confirmed by both *in vivo* and post-mortem analyses. Many implications of that smaller hippocampus have been posited.

This reduction in size of the hippocampus is present at the onset of schizophrenia - suggesting a neurodevelopment explanation of schizophrenia - and worsens as we age. While this happens to everyone, not just to those of us living with schizophrenia, we experience the degeneration to a greater extent and earlier in our lives than those living without schizophrenia. Furthermore, studies have shown that close family members, who do not themselves have schizophrenia, have a smaller hippocampus than would be expected by chance.[60] It is unsurprising, then, that the majority of us who live with schizophrenia have memory impairments, affecting our recall of our pasts as well as our simulations of our futures.

We have, as a group, significant deficits in one particular aspect of memory, our memories of our personal past (autobiographical memory). It concerns what we have lived through - what would be included in an autobiography were such a book written. Having a particularly hard time with autobiographical memory correlates with a smaller hippocampus; a large meta-analysis, involving over 550 participants, found that a moderate to large deficit in this type of memory is common in people

---

[59] Bogerts et al. 1985

[60] e.g., Seidman et al. 1999

with schizophrenia.[61] We are less specific and note fewer details when we recollect a memory than people without schizophrenia. Our difficulties remembering our pasts may be a core feature of the disorder; certainly, it is a major cognitive impairment, one of the many experienced by people living with schizophrenia.

Our memories of the future are also less robust than those of people who do not live with schizophrenia, compromising our sense of continuity over time. This can be quite distressing. For example, I find it hard to project myself into the future, which may be common for people with schizophrenia. Consequently, my loss of autobiographical "memory of the future" may be related to my chronic suicidality: I'm having trouble seeing myself in the future and interpret this unmooring as impending non-existence. My complex but disrupted autobiographical memory easily loses track of my values and goals, and what it would take to get me to the future. Add this to my sense of having a "black hole on my back" into which most of my present disappears, never to become a true memory. I feel quite lost, and to compensate I rely heavily on photographs and on others' recollections of what we've done, where we've been, and when we did it (and having my memoir published has given me a great source for re-finding memories).

Sadly, many of my clients suffer the double hit of poverty and estrangement from families and long-term friends, which, combined, mean that they

_____

[61] Berna et al. 2016

have very few pictures of themselves. They, such as Miguel, do not have many - if any - photos to document their childhood, and some do not have pictures of themselves in the present day. I therefore sometimes take pictures on my work phone of my clients on their "good" days, printing them out and offering them to my clients. I did this for the first time with Miguel this week. A few weeks prior, the day after Miguel's birthday, we had been sitting on a bench in the sun, talking. "You look really good today," I remarked. "Can I take your picture?" He consented, and a couple of weeks later, I handed it to him. Miguel - a non-stop talker (in a good way - he has a lot to say) - was silent for a number of minutes as he examined and contemplated this photo. He smiled at it periodically, nodding his head and murmuring something to himself. He held it up, for better light. He was speechless until he was done, then he remarked:

"That's the best picture anyone's ever taken of me."

It obviously meant a lot to him. I was happy to have given him such a gift. It was one of my most wonderful moments at ACT.

As a group, our clients have experienced fewer "normative" autobiographical events (and hence a lack of photographs of such) in their lives such as weddings (not one of our 70+ clients is married), or raising children (a few clients have had children, but none of our clients have custody of their children). Maybe this is partly responsible for the autobiographical memory loss found by researchers? Their research questions too often rely on asking about such major positive memories. Others have found that people with schizophrenia have a particularly hard time remembering their early adult years - precisely when the disease typically appears.

One study[62] sought to examine the correlations between autobiographical memory and hippocampal size in three groups of people: young people living with schizophrenia, older subjects with the same diagnosis, and older people without a major mental health diagnosis. As expected, those with schizophrenia, whether young or old, had a smaller hippocampus and impaired autobiographical memory when compared to the controls. This could not be explained by the antipsychotics taken by those in the schizophrenia groups, nor by the severity and duration of their illness. There were no major differences between the two schizophrenia groups, suggesting, again, that schizophrenia is not a neurodegenerative disorder like Alzheimer's, but rather a neurodevelopmental one. In all three groups, autobiographical memory ability was correlated with the size of the hippocampus.

For those of us who live with schizophrenia, delusions can grow strangely when accurate remembering falls to the wayside. *Knowing* built on Voices and delusions can overtake even the most rational of people. With an unreasonable set of inputs (to his insula, likely, among other areas) Carlin is actually making, in parts of his PFC, the most rational explanations possible, as does Miguel. Detecting delusion by the one experiencing delusion is very

---

[62] Herold et al. 2015

difficult. This lack of basis in reality has the potential to completely derail someone's mental health. Between delusions and paranoia, amongst memory deficits and hippocampal changes, my clients (and I) who live with schizophrenia find comfort in how the *knowing* explains the resulting oddities of our lives. But for some, these stresses of life loom larger than their coping skills, and necessity and opportunity have led them to use "street" drugs as a means to survive life's inequalities. Addictions often follow, catch up, and overwhelm.

Chapter 5

I Don't Like What I Want: Addictions and Anosognosias

I don't like this anymore. It's not doing anything for me. I don't get high from it anymore; I need it just to feel normal. I want it - I don't want to be dope-sick. But I'm long past liking it.

My client, Reise, was describing his current use of "jib" (crystal methamphetamine, a.k.a., crystal meth, or simply "meth.") While there are many drugs of abuse, I will be focusing on meth in this chapter because it is the one most used by my particular clients. When I first met him a few years ago, Reise was closer to the beginning of his addiction to jib, and things were, by his account, rosier: he liked the effects of his jib. He'd smoke it a couple of times a week, a consistency he maintained for a number of years. He would get high, and then come down, but didn't usually "crash." Instead, the stresses and anxieties of his life would crowd into his mind again, readying him for his next hit a few days later, when funds allowed it. That hit of jib would erase the depression associated with his circumstances (poverty, mental health issues, housing dissatisfaction, unemployment), and the cycle of addiction would continue. In other words, he both *wanted* and *liked* the effects of jib.

Crystal methamphetamine was discovered in 1893 and has become a relatively cheap, quick, and intense drug sought out recreationally. It is a stimulant, giving its users energy and alertness, elevated mood, and a decreased appetite that often leads to pronounced weight loss (though not in Reise's case - he likes his sugary foods enough to cancel out any weight-loss effects of jib). The neurobiology underlying meth's actions includes damage to neurons that use the neurotransmitter serotonin, that "happiness" synaptic molecule. However, meth is more well-known for its toxicity that kills dopamine and norepinephrine neurons, and interferes with glutamate activity. Recall that dopamine and glutamate, as well as serotonin, are among those heavily affected in schizophrenia; add meth + schizophrenia and it is a scary combination.

Research suggests that, compared to the norm, there are more dopamine receptors at work in the brains of those of us who live with schizophrenia;[63] meth keeps more dopamine "swimming in the moat" (by reversing the mechanism that normally allows the presynaptic neurons to "reabsorb" - reuptake - the dopamine after a release). They therefore potentiate each other: more dopamine (from the meth) + more

---

[63] Wong 1986

receptors (from schizophrenia). Could this lead to a more intense high from meth in people with schizophrenia, putting them at greater risk of permanent damage to their brains - or both?

In the early days of his affair with jib, Reise enjoyed the high - a rush that Miguel described once as "a trip to the moon!" Reise was not ready to stop, even though his use drained the small funds he received monthly from the government (he, like most of our clients, collects "PWD" - Persons With Disability - cheques; I too received PWD for one particularly low period of my life). Rent comes off automatically, before it reaches the pockets of the recipients (a wise move), so he did not have to fear for his housing. Thus, Reise settled into a routine of spending his money on jib, cigarettes, and coffee.

I went to see Reise once a week, on Tuesdays, and he would invariably be waiting for me on the patio in front of his building. The large "home" style living arrangement was a suitable place to live. It is on a quiet street lined with sweeping trees, and the houses are neat, with flowers in their beds; there is often the smell of mown grass. Reise's bachelor suite has its own kitchen corner and, surprisingly for mental health subsidized housing, a tub in the private bathroom. Other residents had obvious difficulties with their mental health issues, a prerequisite for living at this housing complex. Staff were engaging and involved and had established relationships with our ACT team to better support clients such as Reise.

Reise and I would talk about his use and he expressed faith in his ability to stop: "When I want to stop, when I'm ready, I will," he said to me, repeatedly. "I've done it before with crack cocaine and alcohol and gambling." Indeed he has done this, and well. I commend him, then push him a bit.

"Was it a sort of substitution? Replacing alcohol with crack, and then crack with jib, for example?" I ask.

"I guess so."

"So what will you replace jib with? As long as there's nothing filling the place of the jib, it will stay." Reise's thought remained undeterred: he would stop when ready, and he wasn't ready yet. Jib was still something he both liked and wanted.

That doublet - liking and wanting - is the subject of current theories on addiction, and is thought to relate to pleasure and desire, respectively. This dichotomy, observed in the 1990's and remaining current in research paradigms, is known as the *incentive sensitization* theory of drug use and abuse.[64] Here, what the person likes is dependent on endogenous opioids and endocannabinoids in specific subcortical areas ("hedonic hot spots" in some mesolimbic structures, such as the nucleus accumbens and ventral pallidum).[65] Throughout these mesolimbic areas - and therefore in some overlap with the "hot spots" of liking - the brain's "reward circuits" use dopamine to drive the wanting.[66] This doesn't mean that you "like heroin (an opioid) and want crystal meth." Rather, any drug - or any substance (drug, food) or activity (gambling, sex, shopping) - draws you towards it with how much

---

[64] Robinson and Berridge 1993; Robinson et al. 2015
[65] Berridge and Robinson 2003; Berridge et al. 2010
[66] Robinson et al. 2015

you like it (in the opioid "hot spots") while creating in you a feeling of wanting more (in the dopamine mesolimbic area reward circuit).

In the beginning, you may like the feelings of being high, as endogenous opioids surge in your "hot spots." As you pass from use to deeper abuse, pleasure can become minimal, and you may look for your next hit even while you're taking the one right in front of you. Your reward circuit invariably makes you crave your drug of choice: a strong, physiological want of *more*. Reise thus uses more jib, but it is with less hedonic impact; withdrawal comes sooner after he uses than it did formerly. "I need it just to feel normal," he stated repeatedly as his addiction grew. At first, drugs pull you, entice you towards them with hedonic reward and you like them; later the addiction kicks you as you stumble in search of the very thing you no longer like. Enjoyment has fled. Addiction has arrived.

With his jib, there was plenty fodder here for Reise's opioid and dopamine pathways. At first, his brain centres and networks said to him, *"This is good. More of this, please!"* As this liking turned to bare dopamine wanting, I wondered if schizophrenia's apparent excess of dopamine makes drug addiction that much harder to stop (*"This is even more rewarding!"*), or whether antipsychotics, with their dopamine dampening, would prompt higher use (*"We need more dopamine!"*). Does the brain search for optimal levels of dopamine?

Regardless, the high jib offers come with another price. It is not uncommon that, particularly for people such as Reise who have a brain diagnosed with a psychotic disorder (e.g., schizophrenia), meth can induce psychosis, perhaps by its influence on the dopamine system. This may increase hallucinations, delusions, and paranoia. It is why we sometimes are at a loss to tell whether a client has an underlying brain disorder (in most of our cases, schizophrenia is suspected) or simply has too much meth in their system.

A drug-induced psychosis can be transient, or may persist even in the absence of acute drug use. Both can look very similar to "regular" schizophrenia. When we at ACT are at a loss to diagnose between these possibilities, and the client's behaviour suggests a psychosis, we may admit them to the hospital. Usually, though not always (some visitors are crafty in smuggling drugs in for the inpatient), this allows the meth to clear from their system and thus give us a clue as to the cause of their presenting psychosis. If they "clear," the hospital will discharge promptly, and we encourage treatment options for drug dependency; if their psychosis persists, we look at their psychiatric treatment regime (i.e., meds).

It ultimately doesn't matter whether, in the latter case, the psychosis is due to a pre-existing mental illness or to a history of drug use. Either way, the brain is damaged and needs some neurochemical help. If it is likely that they have experienced permanent drug-induced brain damage, their "baseline" has shifted; their brains have changed. At times, I curse crystal methamphetamine and my heart aches when a client says, as one client did, "Meth is my best friend." Sadly, I have seen clients who had once functioned well, living independently and happy with life, but whose meth use later prompted psychosis to the point of eviction and other negative outcomes. Of note, many psychotic meth users direct their anger and blame on the antipsychotics, not their meth, for the ills in their lives.

I am not sick!

Reise's story reminds me of *anosognosia*, that lack of insight brought on by brain damage, either from a neurological/psychiatric illness and/or drug use that has physically changed the brain (such as by the neurotoxic effects of meth). Anosognosia is the physiological inability to have the insight that you are experiencing an illness, with its concomitant redirection of blame anywhere but the disease. Literally, anosognosia is "a" (not) "nosos" (disease) and "gnosis" (to know): the not-knowing disease. It is historically restricted to neurology, but given the blurring line between neurology and psychiatry, as well as the loss of distinction between mental illness and addiction, I am among the many who use the term in cases of psychiatric lack of insight. In fact, researchers have found that 57% - 98% of people with schizophrenia display signs of anosognosia.[67] The patients are unaware they have an illness and do not realize the symptoms of the disease; they then deny that they need treatment. Quite logical, really: treatment is for the ill, and they truly believe that they are not ill; ergo, they do not need treatment.

Anosognosia is physiological; it is not "behavioural" or being "in denial" or "stubborn."

---

[67] Lehrer and Lorenz 2014

Anosognosia in schizophrenia may be linked to problems in the parietal lobes of the brain, specifically at the junction between those lobes and the temporal and frontal lobes, cortical areas involved in synchronizing lots of various inputs from other areas of the brain. Note that, interestingly, this area is very close to the insula (where, remember, there is attempted integration of the internal and the external), which has itself also been linked to anosognosia via "error awareness;" the PFC is also involved.[68]

This "not-knowing disease" likely underlies many involuntary admissions to hospital. How would you understand others telling you that they are taking you to the hospital, when you cannot see your own illness? Personal evaluation by self-reflection does not work when you are anosognostic. Moreover, it makes you over-confidant, utterly convinced by your belief that you are not ill. Alternate explanations are not appraised. Problems with metacognition also go hand-in-hand with schizophrenia's cognitive deficits, compounding the lack of insight.

Hence the tendency for some people with schizophrenia to blame everything on the meds we give them, and not on their drug use, even though it is very clear to us, their treatment team, that it is the street drug abuse that is harming their bodies and lives. A client told me once, about meth: "It's the best thing that ever happened to me." Concerning the psychiatric medication, we have heard: "I'm fine! I

---

[68] Klein et al. 2007

don't need your damn pills! Go the fuck away!" Doctor's orders - the daily pills, the monthly injections - would help much more, if it weren't for the meth. We see it clearly, reliably. Why can't they?

Addiction has been correlated to a loss of the brain's important grey matter (where synaptic connections are made) and white matter (the insulated axons connecting brain areas) that can show up on an MRI scan. For those who have used heavily, areas crucial for memory (the hippocampus) may shrink, and the cingulate cortex (recall that the ACC, or anterior cingulate cortex, is implicated in the salience network) can lose cellular volume as well.[69]

My clients do not know this, and even if they did, they might not care enough to change their use. After all, many users in Vancouver's DTES (and, of course, elsewhere) have not stopped using during the pressing "opioid epidemic." Fentanyl, an extremely potent (read: deadly) opioid, has been found contaminating not just the expected opioid drugs (heroin, morphine, oxycodone, etc.) but others, including meth, as well. The risks of using have multiplied, and many users have lost friends, family, and co-residents to overdose. Miguel counts his losses in the multiple dozens. I worried about Reise, about the risk of using and, in his case, using unsafely: alone, in large doses, and from a wide variety of sources.

Reise does not have a "using buddy" to look out for him, nor a friend with a Narcan kit; Narcan (generic name: naloxone) is an injectable opioid

---

[69] Nakama et al. 2011

antagonist that plugs up the receptors better than the opioid drugs (e.g., fentanyl) can open them. When naloxone is present, fentanyl can no longer get in the receptors, and is thus rendered impotent. In this manner, naloxone reverses an opioid overdose, though this is short-lived, about five minutes. Our Narcan kits therefore contain three doses, giving just enough time for an ambulance to arrive. We at ACT are trained in naloxone administration (we practiced on oranges, being told that piercing human skin with a needle is similar to doing so through an orange's peel) and carry it on us during outreach. We have trained many of our clients and given them as many kits as they request, for free. Naloxone has saved many lives in the DTES, and other places, but beware: the person whose life you just saved may awake angry: "You ruined my high!" As scary as it is, some clients even seek out fentanyl for its "better high."

When you no longer "like"

It didn't last. The liking, that is.

The good news for Reise is that he found employment; the bad news was that it paid well. (He was earning more per week than I was.) Why was this bad news? Reise tended strongly to use according to his means. So while he had hopes of saving some money, it all too easily diverted to increase his use of jib. He used more, then needed more. He began using every day, every morning before work, every evening when he got home.

The "liking" of the high disappeared and the "need" of dependence had overtaken Reise. His physical appearance seemed to mirror his decline; he looked ragged, unkempt, and had lost a lot of weight. *A ghost of himself* - this common phrase became common for Reise. Thus, the bad news was that his drug use was spiraling out of control; and the good news? His drug use was spiraling out of control. Finally, after a few months of the job-money-jib pattern, Reise came to me:

"I can't do this anymore. I need to be in some sort of treatment."

He described his use. Now, instead of refraining from use before work, Reise needed a hit of jib before work, to "get me going." "I don't enjoy it anymore," he said. As the need rose, the liking went down. Soon, while he worked, washing dishes and doing other kitchen tasks, his body and brain would demand more jib, and, when denied, threw Reise into withdrawal. Moans of dope-sickness escaped at work, and his boss became aware. Soon thereafter, he was laid off, but the employer was compassionate: "If you get treatment, I'll hire you back."

Suddenly, Reise was without the extra income and was facing withdrawal. He now had the valuable insight that jib had taken over his life. He freely acknowledged that it had become unmanageable. His "managing" now included some small-time dealing, and he became unnaturally aggressive towards those who delayed in their payments. His brain screamed for more jib; he yelled at his customers for more money. Reise's building manager got in touch with me, telling me all of this. Threat of eviction followed.

Yet when my colleague, Ulysses, and I presented these concerns to him, Reise downplayed, minimized, and dismissed it all. In contrast to the desire to go to treatment at "Everrest," which he did re-affirm at every visit, he bestowed on Everrest an almost magical ability to cure him of his woes. It was Everrest, and nothing else. He may have shown the insight to want treatment (defying anosognosia), but seemed unfocused, unwilling to try any other supports.

"Naw," Reise told us in his easy accent. My colleague and I were at Reise's home with ramped up concern and practical steps Reise could take while waiting for a bed in the treatment centre he had chosen. "I won't go to detox. I'll wait for the treatment. It worked last time." He began minimizing his circumstances. "I'm not dealing. People just come to me and ask, and I give it to them. If they have $10, I take it. But they ask me." Housing at risk: "I stopped doing it when the manager told me to." The manager, however, had told me that this was not so. Reise continued to minimize and look to Everrest as the panacea, as if he was thinking, *no need to start until there*. Ulysses and I left him with a copy of the Daytox group schedule, which he accepted, but without commitment to attend.

Why the magical thinking? No matter; it worked. He got there, to Everrest, admitted in place of someone who decided at the last minute not to attend. We at ACT heard nothing of his progress over the next few weeks, but were glad to have seen him go. Then, the local hospital phoned: Reise had been admitted for extremely high blood-sugar levels (in the 40's when ideally we should test at around 6) and the related diabetes. Treatment at Everrest was put on hold till the next intake; Reise was back in Vancouver.

He had lost weight and needed to test his sugars often. At first, he said that he felt "great" - better than he had ever been when "sugared." He was making changes in his diet: no more cakes and pies and pop from the Safeway grocery store he used to frequent. This momentum ought to have continued, but as Reise returned to the jib, he lapsed in his monitoring and let more sugar in. He'd tell me this, with a chuckle of not really believing it all. Realities were not sinking in.

Sugar, sugar, and baby neurons

Reise's relationship with sugar reminded me of the gut's abundance of neurons. Remember the "neural highway" vagus nerve running between the brain and the "gut's brain" (that we saw earlier in the context of *knowing*)? More sugar in Reise's diet meant more sugar wreaking havoc in his gut. If the sugars remain high, as they do in Reise, serotonin and dopamine circuits, among others, change, and not for the better. For one, sugar suppresses the activity of BDNF (brain-derived neurotrophic factor), one of the brain's main neurotrophins. These are growth factor proteins: they tell "baby" cells to survive, become neurons, and grow. They keep mature neurons and their synapses alive in the face of stress. BDNF goes to work on the postsynaptic neuronal sites, on their dendrites. In the absence of BDNF, NMDA receptors - the very ones we've already seen in the context of neuronal learning and memory - are affected, and it all becomes even more worrisome.[70] Less NMDA

---

[70] Xu et al. 2006

receptor activity leads to the inhibition of GABA's interneuron inhibition. Inhibition + inhibition = a neuron that is more likely to be excited and become active. This is a common phenomenon in the brain. What does all this lead to? Cognitive challenges, just like those we see in schizophrenia.[71]

In fact, BDNF is critically low in schizophrenia.[72] This may be related to the neurodevelopmental origins of this disease, which are thought to culminate in the observed symptoms of schizophrenia, including cognitive deficits.[73] Among those who live with schizophrenia, there is a correlation between BDNF levels and abilities to reason and problem-solve.[74] This may mean that the lower BDNF levels found in people with chronic schizophrenia generally may be associated with their compromised cognitive functions. The cognitive areas of concern include attention and memory, which fit with the findings that BDNF is particularly low in the hippocampus[75] and PFC[76] of people with schizophrenia, precisely where NMDA receptor dysfunction may be going on. However, if we were to do some cognitive training, our BDNF levels might rise, which in turn would help cognition, which would raise BDNF levels.... The perfect upward-spiral set-up.

However, I must add that all this is

---

[71] Zhan et al. 2012

[72] Jindal et al. 2010

[73] Angelucci, Brenè, and Mathé 2005

[74] Ahmed et al. 2015

[75] Rizos et al. 2011

[76] Weickert et al. 2003

correlational; less BDNF and poorer cognitive function may be both related to a more general deficit. Perhaps high stress levels, such as often occur when one is living with schizophrenia; for some, such as Reise with his diabetes, sugar may be to blame. Many, if not most, studies also did not take into account medication, both in the past and at the time of the investigation. All this simply highlights the complex nature of schizophrenia and the limitations of studies that attempt to tease its neurobiology apart. However, there are other enticing finds, such as the finding that if you eat a low-calorie diet, your BDNF levels just might go up.[77] But try to make a pill to increase your BDNF levels and you will be frustrated, because BDNF does not readily cross the blood-brain barrier. (Exercise might help - though isn't it always advised for virtually any disorder and for mental wellness in anyone, regardless of their psychiatric state?)

If and when...

Back to Reise, treatment, and his diabetes. While he acknowledged that he had gotten something out of his brief treatment at Everrest, Reise was reluctant to return. Ulysses and I at ACT tried to convince him, but got nowhere. Then, a perfect day to go to Vancouver's Stanley Park presented itself and a long-awaited promise of a bus trip and lunch there was realized. Between the bussing, lunch (fish and chips for both of us), and walking along the Seawall, Reise and I spent four hours together. I had decided not to use this outing for cajoling and persuading

---

[77] Araya et al. 2008

regarding treatment, and we both relaxed. We did talk of treatment, as Reise brought up the subject, and I noticed that, even without (or perhaps because of) the unpressured atmosphere, Reise went from saying, at the beginning of the outing, *"If* I go to treatment..." to *"When* I go to treatment..." by the end of our afternoon out. This change solidified, and he is currently waiting for the next intake date. Previous objections and excuses ("I need $1,000 to go - for cigarettes and eating out with everyone.") have fallen by the wayside. "I like feeling straight," he emphasizes, both with a look to the time before jib and to a future likewise free of the substance, and I think things will go well for him. I hope.

The futility of treatment?

I was once very, very naive about drug use, addiction, and treatment. Surely if the user simply went to treatment, the habit could be kicked. Working at ACT, though, has widened my perspective. "I could go to treatment, get off the dope," Miguel once explained, referring to his use of crystal meth. "I could do it. But then what? Do I come back here?" he asked, making reference to his living situation. He lives in a building of many users and a few dealers; his friends, neighbours, and acquaintances use. Miguel's generous nature with the people in his life often is repaid to him in free dope: "Just because you're Miguel." Knowing Miguel, I can see why that happens. Other times, Miguel seeks out his dope, and, given his multiple connections both within his building and beyond, it isn't hard to find. Prep, needle, moon. In his apartment, it seems inevitable, even for the strongest of "treated" users. An unchanged environment, with its triggers and sources, is probably the best predictor of post-treatment relapse, and Miguel knows this. I don't have a solution.

Reise and Miguel have shown good insight into their drug use patterns, but this is not always the case. Just as many of our clients lack insight to their mental illnesses, so also with their use of recreational substances. They may be anosognostic to the extent of their use and its impact on their brains and lives. It is not uncommon for our clients to get things backwards, as we've seen before: they blame the medication that we give them (i.e., antipsychotics) for their difficulties and attribute any well-being to their use of street drugs. The disease of addiction demands reasons, however true or false, for continued use.

Reasons, but no excuse

Everything we do - positive or negative - we do for compelling reasons; otherwise, why would we do them? Past experiences beyond our control may predispose us to addiction, and present circumstances may provide a vacuum devoid of other rewards and supports. We might not have had a fully supportive home growing up, or, worse, an abusive or neglectful upbringing. We could have lost positive relationships with friends; lacked job skills or been unable to work for other reasons; been forced into substandard housing or even homelessness thanks to meagre PWD income; and have "fallen through the cracks." We might have had every possible strike against us, and we could therefore have a plethora of reasons for turning to drug addiction. Every reason - but no excuse.

If anyone had an excuse to plead "excuse" it would be Aaron. The reasons for his drug use began even before he was born, with intergenerational traumas abundant. In this supposed multicultural country, the Canadian government has explicitly and with force taken Indigenous children away from their families, languages, and cultural practices and deposited them in residential schools. There, a multitude of abuses were rampant. These schools operated for generations (1870's - 1996) and their harms will continue for generations more. Significant racism and a deep lack of support from "systems" continue; Vancouver's DTES population is greatly skewed, with a much higher percentage of Indigenous residents than there is in Vancouver generally. All these abuses that Aaron has faced pointed him in the direction of poverty, substandard housing, and addiction. How could he not be taken by heroin, that "warm, strong hug"?

The Aaron I saw in my first months at ACT had been ravaged by his drug use. Infection in his hip had him bent over in a wheelchair and he lived in a horrendous SRO hotel. Yet, there was *something* in Aaron that refused to be extinguished. His reasons for his heroin addiction were many, but he ultimately refused to let those reasons become excuses. Aaron felt he could trust us at ACT to be a good thing in his life; for the first time in quite a while, Aaron saw that someone believed in him. With time, Aaron asked to be referred to a treatment centre based on Native (to use the term Aaron uses) principles and practices. The process of application was long and at times frustrating, but about a year ago, Aaron arrived. Unfortunately, he had used too much heroin too close to his admission day, and he ended in hospital for severe withdrawal. He had hoped he'd have been able to "tough it out" unnoticed, but his body was vulnerable, and he had to return to Vancouver.

Another reason. But, Aaron still knew in his heart that there were no excuses, and he tried again at the next intake. I volunteered to accompany Aaron, and we set off to the ferry. Aaron was visibly full of hope; he'd been clean for a month or so, and, having received that first glimpse of the program, was highly motivated. Six weeks later, I again travelled to Vancouver Island, to accompany Aaron home. I had felt highly honoured when he had invited me to attend his graduation and I was moved to tears at the ceremony: at his turn to speak, he said, "I love myself now." The heartbeat of the drumming, the strong bonds between the men, and a delicious salmon dinner were altogether overwhelmingly *good*. Aaron smiled the entire time.

He had put his all into those weeks and now the test: returning home. But it wasn't home to the DTES SRO; I had promised Aaron when I left him at the centre that I would "do everything in my power to find you proper housing." When, a few weeks before Aaron was due home, a suite at a recovery-oriented building came to our attention at ACT, I advocated for Aaron to get it. After yet another referral on my part and a sobriety plan on Aaron's side, he moved in. He never even set foot in his old place; we had moved his belongings earlier for him. It was a fresh start, and Aaron was fiercely determined to discover his new life. Addressing the reasons he formerly used, he had faced the "no excuse" squarely. Now, that almost-hidden spark I'd seen before was burning full-flame.

I've heard it said that "the opposite of addiction is not abstinence; the opposite of addiction is connection" and I believe this is powerfully true. Aaron is living it: he connects to people, whether individually or in groups such as the Talking Circle and sweats he attends. He is connected to ACT: Mondays he frequents our Monday Wellness Group (built on principles of DBT, dialectical behavioural therapy) and then we visit for half an hour or so. Aaron describes the rituals (smudging, meditation, affirmations, etc.) that he connects with to keep his positive attitude. We talk of the challenges, too, such as getting irritated and angry when he can't sleep at night because his neighbour is too loud. He has gone through the "12 steps" and beyond. He connects with his Native community and calls home often. I can hardly go out with him without him greeting someone along the way. His addiction is so far from him: he has successfully connected elsewhere. He just can't seem to stop smiling.

Chapter 6

Coffee and a Cigarette

I'm not a member of the club, but I know the secret handshake: it's the morning coffee, with a cigarette. I have never inhaled nicotine from a cigarette, and average one coffee per week at the most; I have no first-hand experience of the combination. I've certainly heard about it, though, and it piqued my curiosity: what is the neuroscience of this magical duo?

Given my diagnosis of schizophrenia, I am, as a non-smoker, in the minority. I've heard estimates of how many people with schizophrenia smoke cigarettes to be about 88%[78] - a huge difference compared to the overall population (estimated at about 15% of the adult population in Canada). Most of my clients smoke and all imbibe caffeine. While I am firm in not buying my clients cigarettes, I must admit my contribution to their caffeine intake, as most of my visits with my clients are held over an

---

[78] Els et al. 2011

ACT-funded cup of coffee. In our society, "let's go for a coffee" has become a euphemism for "let's talk" and since my main role is talking with my clients, I supply the caffeine. Some prefer Tim Horton's; others swear by Starbucks; most will take whatever the closest coffee shop offers. Usually we go together though I have occasionally brought them the cup myself (some of my clients have mobility issues, or one might be in hospital and unable to get a non-hospital "real" coffee). When given the choice between a sweet or a coffee, they will almost invariably choose the latter. They are consistently grateful: $2 for a coffee is actually hard to come by on their limited income, so "my treat" (read: ACT's paying for theirs - but not for mine) is indeed a real treat to them and I know they look forward to it. A simple coffee has smoothed things into a good rapport for many a reluctant and skeptical new client, or for a client who has felt unheard.

For my morning clients, my promise of a coffee gets them up and going. When the weather is not too cold, Carlin opts for coffee to go, as this means he can pair the caffeine with nicotine. We head to the local park, sit on a bench away from those who might object to the smoke. Carlin, like my other clients, is considerate, and we change places on the bench so that the smoke he exhales drifts away from me. I can see him savouring a drag of the smoke and a gulp of the joe. It is what many of our clients crave most when hospitalized involuntarily (i.e., without passes).

It used to be that the locked psych wards had adjoining smoking rooms, where most of the patients spent the majority of their day. When I was a patient at the former Riverview Hospital, cigarettes were doled out by staff, one per client per hour on the hour. When they had finished their smoke, they hung out inhaling the haze of the second-hand smoke that filled the smoking room; ventilation was poor. UBC's smoking room had better circulation, but it still choked me if I went in to pass on a phone message or other such errand. Since those years, the hospitals have cleared out the smoke rooms in the name of health. It makes sense - hospitals have the mandate of promoting wellness over the well-documented physical - deadly - ills of smoking. They now offer nicotine replacement therapies, either patches or cartridges, but these are woefully inadequate for the many heavy smokers among patients with schizophrenia.

"Can you take me out for a smoke?" This is usually the first thing a smoking client says - pleads - to ACT staff when we pay them a visit on the psych ward, where passes may be difficult to come by. Other clients call the office repeatedly: "When is someone coming? I need a smoke!" There are veins of desperation in their pleas. When we can, we do, though we, as employees of a health authority, must not supply the cigarettes themselves - but I am willing to stop as my client asks each person our path crosses: "Do you have a smoke?" Some days are luckier than others for them; sometimes they have a couple of quarters to pay for a cigarette or two. Often, they receive a free smoke from a stranger; fellow smokers are likely compassionate and generous given their own experiences of nicotine craving and withdrawal. In many places, such as a substance use treatment centre or a hospital, cigarettes are the preferred currency and sharing is the ultimate courtesy. Ulmer asks passers-by with an instinctive appraisal of who might be a smoker, and they are usually right.

The caffeinated schizophrenic brain - with sugar?

A coffee is more than just a cigarette's partner. Caffeine, a stimulant, is the number one psychoactive substance used throughout the world. Many cultures, including our own, pair coffee with socializing, and we think nothing of offering a client a large coffee on an outreach visit. Sometimes, it is the only way we manage a short, I-don't-really-want-to-talk-to-you visit with a client. They may brighten with the caffeine, becoming more alert and often more engaged. A craving - today the ACT team comes and takes me for coffee - is satisfied.

Such ingestion of caffeine is highly meaningful, as both common sense and scientific research affirm. After easing the partaker into the day, it structures the rest of the day: the "morning coffee" and a "coffee break" are familiar phrases and rituals. Coffee (and, to a lesser degree, tea) offer the hit of caffeine, and a sugared caffeination is generally preferred. One of our clients, Ellen, insists on 13 sugars in her coffee. In a health-conscious attempt to address this, we suggested a sugar substitute. Thereafter, she took her coffee with 13 Splenda... and the 13 sugars. And if we were the ones to add the sugar, reducing it of course, she could certainly tell and chew us out (swear at us) for it.[79] Reise takes his coffee with four sugars, despite his diabetes; Carlin takes six. There is evidence that sugar could be considered a "drug" itself, and one that can interact with caffeine and nicotine, with which it is often paired.

Indeed, there is some evidence that "you are what you eat," referring to a diet high in refined sugars that doesn't do anyone - particularly those living with schizophrenia - any good. Specifically, the consumption of high levels of refined sugar (and dairy products) could foretell who would be worse off two years later, psychiatrically speaking.[80] The results of consuming a lot of sugar are not unlike those we saw about addictive drugs, such as meth, in the last chapter. Sugar spikes dopamine in the same places (most notably the mesolimbic dopamine reward pathway[81]) as meth, cocaine, opioids, and nicotine do. Furthermore, the intense cravings for sugar rival those for other drugs.

Self-medication?

The most common explanatory reaction to any question of substance use (here, caffeine, and later, we will see, nicotine; sugar, too?) is self-medication. Many of my clients, despite adherence to their prescribed medications, continue to suffer symptoms. Carlin is generally agreeable to taking his antipsychotic injection every couple of weeks, but, despite the psychiatrist's jiggling of which

---

[79] Sadly, Ellen has since died.
[80] Peet 2004
[81] Shariff 2016

antipsychotic is used and at what dose and/or frequency, he lives with symptoms of his mental illness. Would Carlin be suffering even more were he to curtail his high intake of caffeine? (One morning I arrived to take him for a coffee and a visit... "Sure," he replied, then proceeded to tell me that he'd already had six!) Reise, too, drinks caffeine as often as financially possible. Are Reise and Carlin subconsciously addressing their symptoms with an excess of caffeine?

On the other hand, my clients may be trying to offset not the schizophrenia, but the side effects of the pharmaceuticals that they are taking. The prescribed antipsychotics are often very "dirty": they have a range of side effects, from minor to severe, because they attach to receptors in both areas relevant to treating schizophrenia (yay) and areas that are not relevant to schizophrenia (darn). For example, antipsychotics generally suppress synaptic use of dopamine: in the PFC, they alleviate symptoms of schizophrenia such as delusions and paranoia, while in the substantia nigra, less dopamine activity means the tremors, rigidity, and shuffling gait of parkinsonism (side effects that are very similar to the symptoms of Parkinson's disease). Given that staff at Thomas's housing notice that his shuffle to the coffee pot first thing in the morning is more pronounced than later in the day, I wonder if he is relying on the caffeine (and the nicotine he pairs it with) to unofficially treat the reduced gait length his clozapine initiates. Drug development is increasingly focused on tweaking meds to make them more specific (e.g., to a receptor subtype) so as to result in more efficacy and fewer side effects. If indeed caffeine (and nicotine) are being used to address side effects of antipsychotics, would this mean that people with schizophrenia will use less caffeine (and nicotine) in a future in which antipsychotics are, hopefully, much more specialized?

However, there are suggestions in the research that caffeine and the schizophrenic brain do not mix well.[82] This could be problematic, as, compared to the general population, people with a mental illness imbibe more caffeine - and people with schizophrenia do so more than those with a different mental health diagnosis.[83] What is it about the brains of those living with schizophrenia that makes this so, and does this matter psychiatrically?

It seems obvious that the sedation encountered under the influence of most antipsychotics would drive people with medicated schizophrenia to consume caffeinated drinks to increase their alertness. But then, there is good evidence[84] that excessive amounts of caffeine actually exacerbate the schizophrenia itself. The neuroscience of schizophrenia, antipsychotics, and caffeine is complicated. Remember the dopamine hypothesis of schizophrenia? And then the evocation of glutamate as a modulator of dopamine? Now there is another hypothesis: that both dopamine and glutamate are under the spell of caffeine's natural counterpart, *adenosine*. It is a small but mighty molecule that,

---

[82] Thompson et al. 2014

[83] Zimmermann et al. 2012

[84] Thompson et al. 2014

among other roles, influences the activity of dopamine and glutamate circuits. It does this despite being itself a neuromodulator, not a classical neurotransmitter. (That is, for those of you who want the neuroscience, for a bioactive molecule to be considered a neurotransmitter it must be stored in synaptic vesicles, be released by excited presynaptic neurons, and act exclusively at synapses in the nervous system; a neuromodulator, such as the BDNF we've already seen, may act on areas other than the synaptic cleft and may affect either locally or have a more widespread circle of effect.) As a neuromodulator, adenosine has multiple mechanisms of action.[85]

Importantly, caffeine, as an adenosine antagonist, binds to adenosine receptors and renders them useless. This means, according to the above hypothesis, that now both the dopamine and glutamate systems are malfunctioning - a perfect recipe for the molecular and experiential symptoms of schizophrenia. When caffeine blocks adenosine it increases dopamine's power by regulating its presynaptic release *and* affecting responses in the postsynaptic neurons: it gets you coming and going. Meanwhile, the blocking of adenosine by caffeine is also inhibiting glutamate at its infamous NMDA receptors - remember, those receptors that are critically involved in making memories? The take-home message of this is: caffeine means more dopamine and less glutamate are around, just like in schizophrenia.

---

[85] Boison et al. 2012

Given that caffeine, as an adenosine blocker (antagonist), potentiates dopamine and inhibits glutamate, it follows that caffeine ingestion may, at high doses, mimic signs of schizophrenia. Conversely, we might theoretically be able to enhance adenosine's natural abilities (by introducing adenosine receptor agonists, for example, or by finding a way to keep adenosine in the vicinity of the receptors longer); would this act like an antipsychotic medication? If the adenosine theory of schizophrenia is correct, it might. Already, there are clinical studies that support this idea ("overwhelming evidence" says one group of researchers[86]). As yet, there are no such antipsychotic drugs to have been brought to market. Side effects are of concern.

In support of this adenosine hypothesis, postmortem studies of people with schizophrenia[87] have shown that there is a significant increase in the density of adenosine's receptors in this population. If we were able to examine the brains of people with schizophrenia over their lifetime, would we see an ongoing increase? Do we accumulate these receptors gradually over time… with each day that we consume a coffee or two or seven? Often an increase in receptor density means that the neuron is crying out: *"Please give me more adenosine! I've put out extra receptors in hopes of getting a better signal!"*

Caffeine also interferes with GABA,[88] that inhibitory neurotransmitter, which means the

---

[86] Boison et al. 2012

[87] Boison et al. 2012

[88] Ribeiro and Sebastião 2010

glutamate neurons they synapse on are less "excited."[89] Thus, the reduced glutamate activity of schizophrenia is found again.

Jumpy

We commonly know the coffee jitters, that feeling of being a bit "jumpy" after over-consuming caffeine. When we hear a loud noise while well caffeinated, we might jump in surprise: a startle reflex. If we then hear the same noise again, the second startle is weaker. As seen in Chapter 1, this is called prepulse inhibition (PPI) and we experience it in a variety of circumstances. However, people with schizophrenia startle the second time just as much as when the noise was first experienced: they do not display appropriate PPI. Recall Glenn, who jumps at every loud noise? I have seen him startle at a second or third or even fourth noise with just as much strength as the first.

Interestingly, both antipsychotics and molecules that mimic adenosine (agonists) can reverse PPI deficits[90] - though not always. I see with Glenn, who takes the antipsychotic clozapine, that his history of trauma keeps him sensitized. But do we care about the PPI, really? What does being a bit jumpy matter? Well, like many tests in neuroscience, PPI is just a way of measuring something else - something more relevant to our lives. Intact PPI enhances our abilities to disregard the trivial.[91] Things that happen over and

---

[89] Gurpegui et al. 2004

[90] Boisson et al. 2012

[91] Conway 2017

over again usually don't need us to pay attention to them once we've figured them out. Think, for example, of Glenn again. The other day, he and I were sitting waiting for a bus near a construction site. There were several loud noises from the construction, and while we both jumped at the first big bang (haha, pun unintended but appreciated) only Glenn continued to do so for the three or four times it happened. I had received the message, *This is not relevant to my life. I can relax.* Meanwhile, Glenn did not get this check, even when I pointed out the source of the noise and its likelihood of recurring. Now imagine having days full of intrusive stimuli, with impaired physiological calming down. Little wonder Glenn relies on prn's of an anti-anxiety medication. His malfunctioning PPI really makes his life that much more stressful. He worries about startling and falling. Regarding the risks of further PPI impairment, I'm thankful that while he has his two cups of coffee each morning, that's about it for the day. His sensitive system likely couldn't tolerate any more adenosine antagonism from caffeine.

Ethical bean?

Therefore, given the evidence above, should we, as health care professionals, continue to caffeinate our clients? Researchers[92] classified four to seven cups of coffee a day as carrying a "significant health risk" that could exacerbate symptoms of mental illness. Only four cups! That seems all too feasible. Especially when you consider that people with schizophrenia

---

[92] Carey et al. 1999

drink, on average, *seven times* more caffeinated beverages than the average person.[93] I wonder if this may be related to the fact that many people with schizophrenia spend a considerable time in hospital, where there is little to do other than making yourself cup after cup of coffee or tea. But now some wards only provide decaf. I wonder, again: do they have the patients' mental health in mind or are patients "easier to manage" when not stimulated by caffeine? Does this relate to the effects of caffeine on the symptoms of schizophrenia?

I have heard many patients grumble about not getting their coffee fix; however, the louder grumble is about not being able to smoke.

The nicotinic schizophrenic brain

Are you a smoker? Are you feeling drowsy, noting a bit of anxiety, and finding it hard to concentrate - on reading this book, perhaps? Is it difficult to enjoy things that usually bring you pleasure (anhedonia)? If you're a smoker, you may need a cigarette, though whether that smoke will be to self-medicate your schizophrenia or whether you are in a mild withdrawal from your nicotine is hard to tell; the symptoms are similar.

Then, there is a feeling of reward, of pleasure in a smoke. "Reward salience" researchers say, meaning that the good feelings a smoke gives are front-and-centre, something to repeat, and repeat again…. Thomas smokes half a pack a day, while Reise goes through a pack or two. Miguel's smoking

---

[93] Larson and Carey 1998

is touch-and-go, but generally present. As a group, smokers with schizophrenia smoke more per day[94] and they have higher serum levels of the nicotine.[95] I see much of Reise's meager government disability cheques go to funding his habit; if he fits the statistics, and I think he does, he spends upwards of 20-40% of his money on smokes.[96] I can tell when his money runs out each month, as that is when he switches from tailor-made cigarettes to home-made smokes of ZigZag papers and bits of tobacco scraped out of the multitude of butts he resourcefully finds on the sidewalk.

Some powerful addiction is obviously at work; indeed, research suggests that nicotine is as addictive as meth, cocaine, or heroin.[97] Moreover, something about having schizophrenia makes it an even tougher fight. As I've stated earlier, 85-90% of people with schizophrenia smoke. When I consider my clients, I think it is about 90% in that group, and even most of the 10% who don't currently smoke have done so in the past. This rate is even higher than that for any other psychiatric diagnosis. There is something different about the brains of people living with schizophrenia when it encounters nicotine.

For those with a diagnosis of schizophrenia (or schizoaffective disorder), such as Reise and Thomas, their consumption of nicotine may actually be helping their brains (while, admittedly, harming other organs

---

[94] Berg et al. 2015
[95] MacKillop et al. 2011
[96] Kisely 2008
[97] Pontieri et al. 1996

such as their lungs). Many good studies[98] - well-designed "randomized, placebo-controlled, double-blind, crossover" ones - have looked at what nicotine can do for the schizophrenic brain. Or against it... there are conflicting theories.[99] Smoking indeed correlates with the severity of schizophrenic symptoms and poorer outcomes.[100] So, before turning to the neurobiochemistry of nicotine, let's first look at the ways in which it affects smokers at the behavioural level.

Recall that people with schizophrenia can have difficulties filtering relevant information from the irrelevant (PPI deficits contribute to this). The attention needed for tasks lags, learning is hindered, and memory can fail us. Carlin seems distracted, unfocused when I greet him in the morning, but by the time he's taken a few drags on his morning cigarette he is more alert and generally stays "on" for a 45 minute visit. It is not a coincidence: the nicotine in his smoke has reached his brain within a mere ten seconds of his first, long drag. Interestingly, if Carlin is like most people with schizophrenia, he has gotten more nicotine per inhalation than smokers who don't have the diagnosis.[101] In any case, enhanced focus is a well-known result of nicotine, and in people with schizophrenia who smoke, such as Carlin, it is all the more apparent given the cognitive issues often present in this population.

---

[98] Hong et al. 2008; Barr et al. 2008; Jubelt et al. 2008
[99] Berg et al. 2015; Parikh et al. 2016
[100] ibid.
[101] Jubelt et. al. 2008; Berg et al. 2015; Parikh et al. 2016

In people who do not have schizophrenia, certain neurotransmitter receptors (acetylcholine, a.k.a. ACh, which we will encounter soon) habituate to repetitive stimuli. Research[102] has long since found that PPI is normalized not only by the adenosine we saw earlier in this chapter, but is also helped by nicotine. The cognitive impairments common in schizophrenia have more recently come into research and treatment vogue, and these are precisely the ones nicotine appears to alleviate.

Recall that people with schizophrenia have problems in that prepulse inhibition (PPI) situation. When we look at their hippocampus (memory hub, remember? ...if not, that is rather ironic) it is not resting after the pre-pulse of PPI.[103] The repeated, irrelevant sensory stimulations that should not be sent out for further processing by other areas of the brain are kept. Altered, false memories appear, often with significant, special self-importance. They fail to disregard the trivial and instead weave it into their (delusional) thoughts. Things take on an inappropriate personal significance. Instead, For example, as we saw in Chapter 4, Carlin's memories of him moving items in his suite are gone, and his hippocampus has likely mediated false certainties[104] that someone else has moved his things.

Smoking immediately prior to a PPI evaluation can help you perform well.[105] (On the contrary, I wonder: are smokers more "jumpy" when in

---

[102] Hong et al. 2008

[103] Conway 2017

[104] Barr et al. 2008

[105] Hong et al. 2008

withdrawal?) However, acute nicotine abstinence - such as that created by involuntary hospitalizations - can disrupt PPI. PPI is considered a good indicator of the level of dysfunction present in people with schizophrenia. It correlates nicely with how many and strong our baseline symptoms are, and PPI dysfunction is present in family members of people with schizophrenia, though to a lesser degree. All this over-stimulation caused by abnormal PPI (and other "sensory gating" deficits such as latent inhibition... you can look that one up) in schizophrenia may account for the degenerative loss of neurons throughout the brain's more advanced areas (i.e., the cerebral cortex). But nicotine has also been shown to be neuroprotective here: it inhibits the activity of certain specialized cells in the brain (microglia) whose job it is to "eat up" neurons that aren't up to par.[106]

Dear me, it's getting confusing, isn't it?

Working memory, which is our mental space that holds the several pieces of data we are using in any given moment to complete a task (like my trying to keep all these neuroactive molecules straight in my head as I write this!) is bettered by nicotine (darn, I don't smoke), and so is memory in general. Many of these and other cognitive tasks are easier with nicotine in your system as it reduces impulsivity and increases our ability to suppress and/or delay a response.[107] For example, nicotine helps when doing the *Stroop Test* in which you must identify a word's font colour while resisting the strong urge to read the

---

[106] Conway 2017
[107] Barr et al. 2008

word - which is another colour. Think trying to say the colour "blue" when the word reads "RED" or "red" when it says "BLUE." It's frustratingly harder than it sounds! (Get some colouring markers out and try it yourself.) In all this, people with schizophrenia who smoke may be helped by the extra nicotine more than other groups of smokers, perhaps because we who live with schizophrenia are starting, on average, at a lower baseline for tests of our cognitive abilities.

These well-supported indicators that nicotine significantly improves cognitive dysfunction in schizophrenia have led researchers to wonder if they could make a pharmaceutical that acts like nicotine. As always, there is a search for "a pill." This is particularly important, given that as of yet, most antipsychotics do not address cognitive deficits. But even the 30-plus years of research that indicate therapeutic value of nicotine-like substances (i.e., those that can unlock certain neurotransmitter receptors) have not found a suitable medication; they are all too "dirty," working elsewhere and producing excessive and dangerous side effects.

That leads us to the neuroscience of nicotine and other related compounds. Reise takes a drag: the nicotine in his cigarette races into his brain in seconds, having soared unhindered through the blood-brain barrier, and begins its work. It encounters a neurotransmitter system we have yet to look at: that of acetylcholine (ACh). There are two types of ACh receptors and unsurprisingly we will only concern ourselves with the "nicotinic" ACh receptors (nACh). Yes, *nicotinic* ACh receptors let *nicotine* attach just like its natural cousin, acetylcholine. Either way, acetylcholine or nicotine, the receptors open and an ionic charge rushes through with a shot of positive electric charge, making the next neurons more likely to fire action potentials of their own.

Those next neurons to fire may utilize norepinephrine, epinephrine, serotonin, or endorphins, though they are best known for their influence on the dopamine and glutamate systems... hmmm... didn't we just say that about adenosine? As we have seen with Reise, Aaron, and others about their experiences with addiction, dopamine regulation concerns itself with pleasure and is that "reward salience" that links the smoking behaviour with the hedonic feelings. Dopamine activity makes the smoke simply *feel good*.

Dopamine also helps motor control and I wonder if Carlin's slight tremor in his hand is actually less pronounced than it would be if he didn't smoke. Tremors and other motor issues (rigidity, and the shorter gait length Thomas displays) are the parkinsonian side effects of antipsychotics we have examined already. Most antipsychotics induce it to some degree. In parkinsonism (and the related but diagnostically and etiologically different disease known as Parkinson's disease) dopamine neurons (in the substantia nigra) die off.[108] Antipsychotics dampen dopamine neurons elsewhere to achieve their antipsychotic effects, but because they are "dirty" they affect the substantia nigra as well. Thus, parkinsonism as a side effect. Moreover, like people with schizophrenia, more people with Parkinson's

---

[108] Damier et al. 1999

smoke than you'd expect.[109] Are both groups self-medicating?

Then, there's the effects on glutamate, a neurotransmitter that is, as we have seen, affected in schizophrenia and figures prominently in the memory hub, the hippocampus. There, decisions are made about incoming stimuli: *Is this a novelty? Have I seen this before, and, if so, how recently? Should I disregard this - has it happened before with no ill effects? - or should I send it for further processing?* These questions are the crux of sensory gating, such as prepulse inhibition (PPI) that we recently examined. In schizophrenia, these loops go into overdrive and everything seems salient, while neurons begin to die off due to overstimulation. Does nicotine moderate this? In people who don't have schizophrenia there is the endogenous ACh to keep things balanced. In people with schizophrenia, though, there is "abundant evidence"[110] that our nACh system is not functioning properly.

But given all this evidence of nicotine's wonders, we still can't ethically support our clients' smoking. Smoking tobacco is the number one cause of morbidity and death in psychiatric settings. This is due primarily to the lung cancers and cardiovascular diseases that smoking causes. I worry about my clients' lungs especially, such as when 71-year-old Thomas expels a raspy cough or when 60-something Ulmer can't stop coughing. They've both spent time in hospital recently, which amounts to an imposed

---

[109] Morens et al. 1995
[110] Barr et al. 2008

smoking cessation program... at least till they are well enough to get out on passes. Thomas accepts the nicotine cartridges from the nurses as NRT (nicotine replacement therapy), which he keeps inside his mouth instead of inhaling through them. Ulmer just goes without, but calls us at ACT repeatedly to "come take me out for a smoke!"

This request/demand is the most common thing we hear from hospitalized clients. This is not surprising: withdrawal from nicotine has been reported to be harder on people with schizophrenia than on smokers without this disorder. Reise, for example, was provoked to want to leave the recovery program he was in for his addiction to "jib" when he ran out of smokes, despite his determination to "get help." He was experiencing the intense anxiety, irritability, impulsivity, and cravings that accompany nicotine withdrawal, and it was eclipsing all else. His nACh system was crying out for the nicotine it was used to relying on, while his brain was also also missing the jib. Surely two assaults that both culminate in frustrated dopamine reward pathways would be very hard to manage. In this case, the treatment for Reise's life-threatening addiction to crystal meth trumped the importance of quitting smoking; Reise was supplied with cigarettes by the compassionate manager at his housing complex.

It is much harder for people with schizophrenia to quit smoking than those who do not live with this disease; harder, but not impossible, as seen in Glenn, as well as my close friend, Yves. Given that people with schizophrenia who smoke experience a much worse withdrawal when

152

quitting,[111] it is no wonder the addiction to tobacco among the mentally ill is so tenacious. However, the potential benefits are just as compelling: smoking cessation has been linked to less aggression and reduced substance use, so these are behavioural reasons to quit, above and beyond the physical health concerns. Glenn was particularly helped to quit smoking by the medication Champix (generic name varenicline, a partial agonist for a nACh receptor subtype). This medication, prescribed by his psychiatrist, reduced Glenn's cravings and, as Glenn reports, made him feel nauseous at the smell of cigarette smoke.

Personally, I abide by VCH regulations and do not buy cigarettes for a client, not even on their behalf with their money; other members on the team waver on this issue, and sometimes concede, paying out of their own pocket (especially if they themselves smoke/used to smoke). Many will carry a lighter, at least. We generally don't give much thought to our clients' smoking habits, and proceed as if they pale in comparison to the psychiatric treatment they need. Tobacco use is the leading preventable cause of death and disease in the mentally ill. It far exceeds suicide as a significant cause of death amongst those with a mental illness - and we certainly (and rightly) discuss that topic with any client we feel we need to. Why not about smoking?

There is one thing of note about the antipsychotic clozapine, which several of our clients take daily. The effects of nicotine on attention and

---

[111] Parikh et al. 2016

memory are much less robust in those taking clozapine.[112] Also, for active, heavy smokers, such as Reise, higher doses of their antipsychotics may be needed to achieve the same results as those who don't smoke.[113] It makes me wonder if Thomas's sporadic decompensation despite staying on his antipsychotics is related to changes in the number of cigarettes he smokes.

A shared vulnerability?

We've seen evidence that smoking may be how people with schizophrenia deal with cognitive dysfunction: a possible self-medication. This theory is alluring, both in its simplicity and explanatory value. But what if that's not it? A group of researchers,[114] who recently examined 275 articles on smoking, nicotine, and schizophrenia, suggest another theory: the 80-90% of people with schizophrenia who smoke may have a "shared vulnerability." That is, they have something causing both their schizophrenia and their likelihood of being a smoker. The alleviation of cognitive symptoms alone is therefore not thought to be the major motivator.[115] However it works, smoking is often already established before the first episode of psychosis.[116]

Take Reise. He began smoking at 14, thus making him a smoker first, then (later) someone with schizophrenia. Aaron, like Reise, began smoking as a

---

[112] Jubelt et al. 2008
[113] Convey 2017
[114] Parikh et al. 2016
[115] Manzella, Maloney, and Taylor 2015
[116] Smith et al. 2009

young teenager, another example close to the 5.3 years found to separate the onset of smoking and the first episode of psychosis.[117] Why the delay? Was the nicotine increasing dopamine sensitivity, laying the seeds for schizophrenia to grow?[118] After all, daily smokers develop schizophrenia about one year earlier than those who don't smoke.[119]

This age is a period of marked impulsivity, particularly for adolescent boys. Could this precocious impulsivity, particularly their willingness to begin smoking, explain why schizophrenia first appears in young men in their mid- to late-teens while the average age of onset for women (who statistically begin smoking slightly later in adolescence) is their late teens or early twenties? In the time lag between onset of smoking and the appearance of psychosis, nicotine may have been increasing the sensitivity of their dopamine system. Given the role of dopamine in schizophrenia, this could further their vulnerability to this disorder. We really need to study this hypothesis further, ideally with longitudinal studies that can follow these various adolescent events (and genetic vulnerability: do they have close family members with a psychotic disorder? Who smoke?) as the subjects grow from teenagers to adults.

Neither Thomas nor Reise care to try to quit smoking, and in fact Thomas makes a good home-based business selling cheap cigarettes even more cheaply. However, when a customer quits, he is

---

[117] Parikh et al. 2016
[118] Parikh et al. 2016
[119] ibid.

happy (despite his lost business) for their healthy decision. As I mentioned earlier, Glenn used to smoke upwards of a pack a day, but, in his determined manner, has left the nicotine behind. (I wonder, though, if this oral habit morphed into excessive fluid consumption, as he always has a juice or Gatorade or diet drink from crystals to go from cup in hand to mouth. He agrees with this pondering.) It was in some ways harder to quit the smoking of cigarettes than the crack cocaine Glenn also left behind when he decided to, as he says, "turn my life around." There is some suggestion that if we could activate certain subtypes of the nACh receptors, we may facilitate clients' ability to quit,[120] as seen in the role Champix played in Glenn's success.

The caffeinated, nicotinic brain

We've seen the power of the caffeine fix and the draw of nicotine, but what about that magical combination voiced by so many of my clients? Why the "coffee *and* a cigarette"?

Did you notice that, in both the brain's caffeine (adenosine) and nicotine (acetylcholine) circuits, there is a convergence on the dopamine and glutamate systems? Again, we might be missing the point by focusing treatments on altering just dopamine or even just the glutamate levels. Perhaps antipsychotics would be more effective on a variety of positive and negative symptoms, as well as the cognitive ones, if we aimed therapies at adenosine and acetylcholine… just like coffee and a cigarette does. Could we develop

---

[120] Brunzell and McIntosh 2012

medications that hit this combination, while sidestepping the addictive nature of nicotine and, to a lesser degree, caffeine?

Smokers - and remember that 80-90% of people diagnosed with schizophrenia smoke regularly - need two to three times the caffeine to reach the same plasma levels of caffeine as non-smokers.[121] Also, heavy smokers (defined at only 10 or more cigarettes a day!) may need higher doses of antipsychotics.[122] That is, smoking interferes with the metabolism of caffeine (smokers metabolize caffeine faster) and of antipsychotics.[123] So while the nicotine and caffeine may be addressing cognitive and negative symptoms of schizophrenia, they may also be leaving the person with schizophrenia with more positive symptoms (i.e., those best addressed by conventional antipsychotics). It seems like smokers who live with schizophrenia get caught coming and going.

The cycle is circular: smokers consume more coffee and coffee drinkers smoke more cigarettes.[124] Accordingly, heavy smokers drink more caffeine than do non-heavy smokers, and the latter drink coffee more than non-smokers.[125] Caffeine not only works alone; it can greatly increase the pleasure of that paired cigarette such that more cigarettes are then smoked.[126] It is hard to tease out the effects of one over the other and many studies therefore neglect this

---

[121] Gurpegui et al. 2004
[122] ibid.
[123] ibid.
[124] Gurpegui et al. 2004
[125] ibid.
[126] Gasior et al. 2001

confounding variable. Also, it is difficult to control for the pathophysiology of schizophrenia when wanting to compare the ingestion of caffeine or nicotine in both schizophrenic and normal populations. It is interesting that post-mortem studies have found both adenosine receptor levels (as we saw earlier);[127] and nACh receptors[128] to be disordered in people with schizophrenia.

The natural roles of "just-right" amounts of the adenosine (caffeine) and acetylcholine (nicotine) are interesting. In our brains, recall that the PFC concerns itself with the executive functions: regulation of emotion, motivation, and goal-directed behaviours, for example. These can all contribute to the commencement and perpetuation of smoking nicotine and drinking caffeinated beverages. While I would prefer to see my clients content with the adenosine and acetylcholine their brains were designed for, I recognize the need to prioritize. I would think that living in substandard housing, for example, can stress them out and wreak more havoc on their brains and shorten their lifespans to a greater degree than smoking or drinking coffee will. Also, a compassionate peer support worker will have a much more positive impact on them than the potentially negative effects the coffee I provide - and the smoking I tolerate - ever will.

---

[127] Boison et al. 2012
[128] Jubelt et al. 2008

Chapter 7

Why Weight? The Ethics of Clozapine

"She's gaining weight still." She, Elizabeth, had been weighed again recently, and by now her weight gain had surpassed 75+ pounds since she'd started on the antipsychotic clozapine. We were worried about metabolic effects, such as Type II diabetes and cardiovascular disease; she was worried that it was affecting her occupation as a self-identified sex-trade worker, as well as her self-esteem in general.

"But the clozapine, it's holding her. She is so well." That also was true; we had never seen Elizabeth so stable mentally. Which is why we continued to knock on her door, an SRO room in one of the downtown hotels, every single morning, to give Elizabeth her meds:

"Who is it?" we hear through the door, and we announce ourselves: "It's Leah and Erin from ACT." Elizabeth always answers our 10:00am knock, though she takes her own time to rouse.

"It's open."

We push the door inwards, and one of us, the one with the plastic med pouch, enters a few feet into the room. As SROs go, it is relatively large, but much of the space is occupied with things - clothes, mostly, and other items that Elizabeth can't seem to discard. There are two couches, pointing towards the old TV. Elizabeth is on one of the couches, minimally dressed, which only made her weight gain more apparent.

"Here, Elizabeth." Leah tears the pouch, and sprinkles the multicolour pills into Elizabeth's hand. Elizabeth has found a cup, and pours herself some lukewarm root beer. She looks at the pills a moment; she knows what to expect. "This one is for my weight," Elizabeth said once to a friend in the room. She gets 1,000 mg of metformin every morning, which is supposed to at least curtail any further gains.

This is what we were talking about in the meeting that morning. Metformin, a drug marketed as an anti-diabetic medication for Type II diabetes, can halt excessive weight gain, particularly for people who take antipsychotics such as Elizabeth does. We weren't sure whether Elizabeth would benefit from this, or whether it would just be another pill in her hand each morning. It lay, white, beside the colourful clozapine. Clozapine was the culprit calling for our metformin intervention.

Clozapine was, for Elizabeth, effective, in regards to her mental health. Indeed, that is what clozapine promises to most who take it, often working a medicinal miracle to people who have failed to show any significant response to at least two - but often four or more - other antipsychotics. For Elizabeth, antipsychotics x and y and z did nothing substantial. Carefully, we brought out the clozapine; carefully, because it can cause agranulocytosis, a potentially fatal decrease in the body's white blood cells and thus its ability to fend off infections. We walk with Elizabeth a few blocks once a month for the obligatory blood work to monitor for this, thankful that she had so far been in the safe zone. So the clozapine continued... and so did the weight gain.

Researchers are not quite sure the reason behind clozapine's effectiveness where other antipsychotics have failed. Commercially available since 1972, clozapine can be up to twice as effective as other drugs that treat psychosis, including schizophrenia, and is often the only medication that works well for treatment-resistant schizophrenia. It has been thus used since at least the 1980's when it was shown to be superior to chlorpromazine.[129] There is therefore a clear indication that taking clozapine has substantial psychiatric benefits, as we've seen with Elizabeth. But the question remains: when is this benefit eclipsed by the side effects? Increased weight is of note in and of itself, particularly in our weight-phobic culture, and the related toll on the body must be taken into account. We must therefore do the impossible: foretell which would be worse for Elizabeth; which would be best? It pits mental health versus physical health, and prompted us to invite a professional ethicist to our office.

We are back in the morning meeting, aptly "weighing" (excuse me) the options:

"Lifestyle changes, that's what it's got to be,"

---

[129] Kane et al. 1988

insisted Leah. We knew that, all of us did. We all would have liked to change our lives in that way, too. But knowing Elizabeth, and her reliance on heroin, we were very doubtful she would take on a diet and exercise program to lose the pounds she had gained.

"I suppose we could increase the metformin. But giving her 1,500 mg at once when we see her in the morning... It has side effects. Diarrhea." This side effect affects as many as half the people who take metformin, and was of particular worry, given that the SRO hotel in which Elizabeth resides has only one bathroom per floor for the residents... and is situated at the complete opposite end of the hallway to Elizabeth's suite.

Metformin has other effects, too. A side effect that has been seen is that metformin can affect the risk of dementia; according to some studies, susceptibility may decrease cognitive decline...[130] or, increase it, according to others, including a large study involving more than 14,000 patients.[131] Since response to metformin seems at least partly genetic, and vulnerability to dementias can be inherited, this may explain the contradictory findings. Risk of dementias, such as Alzheimer's, here may be a remote consideration, though, considering that, statistically, people with schizophrenia die 12 to 15 years earlier than those who don't have this disease.[132] We - I am included here - simply may not, on average, live long enough to get advanced dementia. Metformin may also stimulate the birth of new neurons in the place in

[130] Ng et al. 2014
[131] Imfeld et al. 2012
[132] Crump et al. 2013

the brain that is most important for memory (the dentate gyrus of the hippocampus), which could relate to its positive effects on certain types of (spatial, hippocampus-dependent) memory.[133] This could potentially counter schizophrenia's negative impact on memory.

Contributing to obesity, cravings for food and subsequent eating binges can dominate in people with schizophrenia taking clozapine, or olanzapine, another antipsychotic.[134] Home meal preparation, which can reduce the calories and processing chemicals that are in ready-made or "fast" or "junk" foods, is problematic: I'm thinking of SRO's, which don't usually house a fridge or even a hotplate. Then there's the higher cost of healthy foods. Together, these mean that healthy eating is a stretch that may be just out of reach for Elizabeth and the many others like her. So was her main hope metformin? Do we increase it, despite its side effects?

"We could ask her which she'd prefer," I offered. Which we did, later that day.

"The pills," was the quick decision Elizabeth made. "I won't get diarrhea." She couldn't see herself eating differently and exercising, no more than we thought she would. We had been at least a bit hopeful that it could happen, and we do continue to offer support in getting exercise; Elizabeth has said that she likes swimming so we bought her a bathing suit and suggested that we swim with her.

That still left us with the question: what if,

---

133 Potts and Lim 2012
134 Kluge et al. 2007

despite the metformin increase, her weight gain continues? "Metformin only stabilizes the weight. It does not affect weight loss," her psychiatrist insisted. I had something to say about that, though. I had mentioned as much to Ulysses before, and he prompted me now: "Erin, you had something to say?"

Blushing, I felt it as a confession to admit to my colleagues that I'd been on metformin for the last year or so. My physician had prescribed it for me for unrelenting weight gain, too: 30 pounds after my first three years at ACT, and it was still climbing steadily. Then, during my first year-long metformin trial, I'd lost about 15 pounds, instead of gaining the usual ten. I took that as a net 25 pounds. Certainly the actual 15 was a "clinically significant" loss (defined as a loss of 7% or more of your body weight). (Since then, I have stayed on the metformin and lost another 15.)

"But that's due to increased activity," the psychiatrist countered.

"No, eating less," I replied, blushing further. She remained unimpressed. She seemed certain that there could be no loss, only stabilization. But, as I read further, I noticed later that, at least in rats, less consumption, not greater levels of activity, is responsible for the weight loss.[135] Eat less, lose weight. Seems straightforward. Though, others[136] suggest its anti-obesity results may be due to less somnolence: if we sleep less, we move more. Likely it is some combination of the two; in Elizabeth's case, her use of

---

[135] Lian et al. 2016

[136] e.g., Barak, Beck, and Albeck 2016

164

"down" kept her dozing much of the day.

I had one more question to raise. "Is betahistine an option? I was reading some papers...." Everyone was quiet, looking at me. Would I ever stop blushing? No comments, then the moment faded. I had been uncertain as to the stage of drug development for the use of betahistine for weight gain, but examined the evidence myself, later, at home. First, it seemed promising, with betahistine being shown to regulate weight in people taking certain antipsychotics, without changing the efficacy of the antipsychotics.[137] Then, I noticed that there is, as with any drug, a whole host of side effects, including nausea, upset stomach, and vomiting. Is that how it is linked to weight loss? You are too nauseous to eat and when you do you may throw up? As I read further, I found a complicated web involving histamine, its various receptors, symptoms of schizophrenia, and regulation of weight.

Antihistamines for schizophrenia?

Given the potential benefits of betahistine in treating weight gain, let's start by looking at histamine and its roles as a neurotransmitter in the brain. The cell bodies of the neurons that release histamine (only 64,000 of them!) are found almost only in a small area of the brain (the tuberomammillary nucleus in the posterior hypothalamus, if you were curious), but they reach out to almost everywhere in the brain. Histamine stimulates the release of other neurotransmitters,

---

[137] Poyurovsky et al. 2005; Lian et al. 2016

including dopamine, serotonin, and norepinephrine. This has me wonder: could this effect of histamine be the cause behind the cause of schizophrenia? That is, we know that in many areas of the brains of those living with schizophrenia there is an overabundance of dopamine; we successfully treat many clients with antipsychotics that lower the dopamine activity. But what if the extra dopamine is actually a result of the lack of histamine? Low histamine activity (e.g., when blocked) may indeed cause dopamine levels to rise.[138] Recall that the theory is that people with schizophrenia have higher levels of dopamine (generally; simplistically)... and, further nailing the case, too little histamine (such as by taking antihistamines) can lead to thought disorders, and hallucinations.[139]

In other words, histamine and dopamine have suspiciously complex interrelations. Dopamine and histamine receptors can operate in the same synapse, and even more compelling is that dopamine receptor parts (subunits) sometimes coexist with histamine receptor parts in the same receptors (as heterodimers).[140] Is histamine's control of dopamine where we ought to be focusing our research and subsequent treatments? What if we used antihistamines instead?

Spoiler: it's been done. First, by a French surgeon who, in 1952, wanted to try the antihistamine chlorpromazine as a medication to reduce "surgical shock" in his patients. When those patients came

---

[138] Dringenberg et al. 1998
[139] Bassett et al. 1996
[140] Ellenbroek 2013

through their surgeries, he noticed that they were more stable mentally. This drew the attention of a psychiatrist, Dr. Pierre Denker, and he started using the antihistamine on his most "difficult" patients. What followed was a revolution in the care of people with severe and treatment-resistant psychotic disorders such as schizophrenia. Chlorpromazine was deemed safe for this population by drug regulators two years later, in 1954. It became the first drug to be used as an antipsychotic. Only ten years later, in 1964, it was being used world-wide - by a staggering 50 million people!

Chlorpromazine may be an antihistamine, but it also blocks dopamine receptors. So which is the antipsychotic action - or is it both? Chlorpromazine is certainly a "dirty" drug: it affects all sorts of the brain's chemicals (besides dopamine and histamine, it also alters the activity of serotonin, adrenaline, and acetylcholine). The dopamine part involves a certain receptor type (the D2 receptor) and it has been since found that the better the D2 involvement, the better the antipsychotic. And so, thus began the search for newer and more specific antipsychotics that focused on dopamine. I think we sort of forgot about the antihistamine part.

Fast forward to today, where we have lots of antipsychotics that zone in on regulating dopamine; indeed, we got so good at getting the dopamine part (Aim 1) right that we then had to start making them interact with other systems (Aim 2), such as the serotonin one, again. Kind of like cell phones: they advanced technology to make them so small (Aim 1) that they then had to make and advertise their smartphones as "bigger is better" (Aim 2). You get too good at one extreme (Aim 1), and you have to totally switch gears (Aim 2).

So... antihistamines? The family members of chlorpromazine drugs are potent, and they haven't been completely forgotten. A few years ago in Finland, in a well-designed study, clinicians found that the drug famotidine, an antihistamine, was better than their placebo for reducing psychotic symptoms.[141] Despite an inkling about famotidine since the 1990's, the studies just aren't there yet for us to go ahead and offer it to Elizabeth.

1, 2, 3 - histamine!

Then, again, there's that clozapine Elizabeth takes faithfully every day, the treatment of our choice for her schizophrenia, after traditional dopamine-focused antipsychotics failed her. Her clozapine "helps out" (an H2 receptor agonist) at some histamine receptors while "hindering" or "plugging up" (an H1 receptor antagonist) at others. Then, things get more complicated. Histamine receptors in the brain come in a variety of flavours, aptly termed H1, H2, H3, and H4. (Note: H4 is not mentioned in schizophrenia-related papers, so we will disregard it here.) There is "helping out" and "hindering" in dizzying combinations and degrees that I will try to make it clear.

First, we will examine the H1 that clozapine "hinders." These receptors are sprinkled throughout our brains, but for those of us with schizophrenia -

---

[141] Meskanen et al. 2013

such as Elizabeth and I - there are generally fewer H1 receptors in our brains, particularly in the front of our brains (frontal cortex). Clozapine (which I have taken as well in the past) "plugs up" the few H1 receptors we have, perhaps contributing to the effects on typical symptoms of psychosis. Treatment for low H1 receptor levels may include a diet high in protein: the amino acid histidine converts to histamine in the body. Should we be bringing Elizabeth some protein bars?

H1 receptor activity also affects our appetites and weight, and are found in brain areas involved in feeding behaviours.[142] The better the drug at "plugging up" the H1 receptors, the more weight is gained.[143] Unfortunately for Elizabeth, clozapine is one of the best at this. Olanzapine, another antipsychotic, has similar effects on both H1 receptors and weight. On the other hand, betahistine "helps" or facilitates (as an agonist) H1 receptor activity.

H2 receptors are "plugged up" (antagonized) by the famotidine we've seen already in the Finnish study; apparently H2 receptor blockade can treat schizophrenia. However, Elizabeth would likely need to take doses five times greater than the standard anti-allergy dose in order to get a statistically significant change in symptoms of her schizophrenia. Such high doses would surely have other side effects.

H3 receptors are interesting, being autoreceptors: receptors on the *pre*synaptic side of the histamine neurons themselves. They are there to slow

---

142 He, Deng, and Huang 2013
143 Kroeze et al. 2003

themselves down: *We just let a whole lot of histamine into the synapse! We should stop sending more!* Yet it still leaves enough histamine around in the synaptic cleft to affect the release of other neurotransmitters in downstream neurons - such as dopamine. That's a clear pathway for antihistamines to act like antipsychotics. Indeed, drugs that "plug up" H3 receptors have antipsychotic effects... in rodents, at least.[144] Shall we check in the pet rats (and not-so-pet rats) in the buildings?

In addition to "plugging up" (antagonism) of H3 receptors as an antipsychotic, antihistamines have a clear role in weight management. By affecting the hypothalamus's feeding areas, H3 receptor antagonism is involved in the how much we eat and the potentially subsequent obesity. It does this by controlling satiety, that feeling of *I've had enough.* Thus, compounds that "plug up" H3 autoreceptors, such as betahistine, could be both anti-psychotic and anti-obesity - just what Elizabeth needs.

When fat cells yell at the brain

Weight gain, whether due to antipsychotic exposure or not, has a lot to do with a hormone called leptin. Fat cells produce leptin in order to tell the brain: *We have enough fat cells! We don't need any more extra calories!* This usually helps us maintain a fairly stable weight over time. But 75% of those who are taking clozapine experience a bigger appetite, and it becomes easy to gain weight. More fat cells, more leptin - but then, the brain (specifically, the

---

[144] Fox et al. 2004

hypothalamus) might not be as sensitive to leptin signals in those who are taking clozapine. Elizabeth might be experiencing an ongoing cycle of feeling the need to eat more all the while not getting a strong leptin signal. Thus, weight gain. She may be trapped in a biochemical perfect storm.

It should be noted that a problem with the majority of the studies on this vicious cycle is that they only cover a matter of weeks. However, they are able to show, statistically, that clozapine causes weight gain. People like Elizabeth, who have been on clozapine a long time, may be experiencing even greater weight gain, perhaps in part via leptin insensitivity. Her mental health has undoubtedly improved; unfortunately, for Elizabeth and for many others, clozapine seems to help most when it also causes more significant weight gain.

It seems there is no easy way out, but there is a population, to which my friend Yves belongs, that intrigues me. Like Elizabeth and I, Yves has been diagnosed with schizophrenia, and he has, for the last decade, taken a daily dose of an antipsychotic. Yves takes olanzapine: 60mg, plus another 10mg as needed each day. That is a substantially high dose, and I would have expected a correspondingly elevated weight, because olanzapine is like clozapine: it usually causes significant weight gain. But Yves surprises me. He is slim. In fact, he notes that he wishes he could gain a few pounds but that he finds that difficult to do. Likewise, there are a few cases reported in which the patients actually lost weight when put on clozapine, even without changing their diet or activity levels.[145] But generally, there is the correlation: the greater the weight loss, the less effective the clozapine is for the psychiatric symptoms.[146] I wonder whether a similar association is true for Yves - that the high levels of the antipsychotic he takes reflect a poorer response to this drug. Interestingly, women (such as Elizabeth) tend to gain more readily than men.[147]

In the end, nothing is straightforward in this area of drugs, weights, and symptoms of schizophrenia. Causes and effects chase each others' weighty tails. But being in a state of mental wellness, such as responding well to an antipsychotic drug, might be a place where you are more able to implement behaviours that help control eating and exercise than when you are psychotic. Without these efforts, cycles of weight gain and related psychological despair may lead to further medication changes... and more weight. What will this do for Elizabeth's quality of life? We are left where we began: ethical considerations of mental versus physical and psychological health, which has a very real application: do we keep bringing Elizabeth clozapine?

[145] Tungaraza 2016
[146] Thomas et al. 2009
[147] Yves, Covell, Weissman, and Essock 2004

Chapter 8

Shaking Hands with the Lonely

The visit is coming to a close. I stand up, pull my bag onto my shoulder, and offer my hand. "Good to see you," I say, looking them in the eye. Their hand closes on mine, and they meet my gaze. "Thanks," they say. The handshake is warm, strong, and I believe that this small ritual means a lot to my clients. Some prefer a fist bump, and I oblige; there is the occasional hug. Either way, I am sending them a clear message: you are seen, valued, and respected; despite our differences, we are peers. It is an acknowledgement that I care about them as a fellow human being. Touching them is a powerful connection.

I think my clients look forward to that handshake that ends our visit. Thomas, Aaron, and Reise all get a little twinkle in their eye when I begin to extend my hand to them; they respond to the strength of my grip with their own. It makes me wonder: how much physical human contact do they get in the rest of their week? When does anyone else in their lives touch them with care? Some of our clients have partners or close friendships, but many are alone. Some cannot stand being touched, and I've been left in an awkward position when I've put out my hand upon meeting a new client, and they have seen it, but rejected it. For some reason, I had not begun this ritual with Miguel, a long-standing client of mine. We part with a quiet "thank you." Part of me wishes I had offered it long ago; it would be so awkward to introduce it now.[148]

Once, though, years ago, Miguel had been certified to the psych ward, and at the end of our first visit on the ward, he asked me for a hug. I obliged, with compassion. Other hugs with different clients have occurred, though I do limit this. The week after Reise returned from his weeks-long stay out of town for treatment (for his use of crystal meth), he looked so lost and unmoored that I felt drawn to say, "Do you need a hug?" I patted his back reassuringly as we hugged. However, when we met again the next week, when he went for a hug, I directed his expression to our usual handshake. Another client, Thomas, asked me for a "birthday hug" which I did give, but politely declined another the following visit. Given the potential of being reprimanded for "inappropriate contact with a client" I try to walk that fine line between human compassion and professional conduct. A handshake serves it well, I think... although once, when another client, Rory, went for a hug and I for a handshake, I narrowly averted a very awkward personal situation.

---

[148] Since then, I did decide to offer Miguel a handshake. It was good, and we now keep the ritual.

A touching story

Touch is a complex sense, with many kinds of neurons doing many different things. It is not, as is the case with much of neuroscience, well understood yet. We are intrigued by this touch, our sense that is our oldest, evolutionarily speaking, and that is our first sense to develop in the womb. Our skin boasts a size of, on average, 18,000 cm^2 if laid out flat, and as such is our largest organ. Touch is more powerful than even our species' claim to fame, our linguistic abilities; it has been said that interpersonal touch is ten times more powerful than language.[149] Touch can directly and instantly affect our emotional well-being. Researchers are actually puzzled at how powerful touch is to us. It has been shown, over and over again, to influence our beliefs and actions even without us being conscious of it. For example, researchers reported that a person is more likely to share a free cigarette with someone else if the person making the request touches the potential cigarette giver.[150] (Should I inform my smoking clients?) One other study[151] had people try to convey feelings (anger, sadness, surprise, etc.) simply by touching the arm of another participant. They were remarkably (though not entirely) able to do this: the touched participants guessed many of the emotions consistently, results that were similar to those of figuring out the emotions from facial expressions.

Touch has also been shown to be vital for

---

[149] Field 2001
[150] Joule and Guéguen 2007
[151] Hertenstein et al. 2006

infant development, both in humans (recall the human-to-human tactile deprivation in under-staffed orphanages that can and has led to significant developmental delays and even, in severe conditions, death) and in monkeys. Harry Harlow, a researcher working in the 1950's, was intrigued by the power of touch, and gave newborn monkeys two "mothers": a wire-mesh one with a bottle of milk, and another covered in fuzzy terry cloth that offered cozy contact but no bottle for the baby monkey. Would the monkey prefer the one who offered nourishment? Not so. The babies would take the bottle, but then return immediately to cuddle on the cloth "mother." If they were afraid, they would invariably cling to the fuzzy, cozy one. They, like humans, had a powerful "touch hunger."[152]

That drive relies on our nervous system's set-up for touch. Touch is sensed in several ways, each with its own type of receptor in the skin, pathways for the nerves headed to the brain, and regions in the brain itself. Think again about that handshake. Most receptors in the skin (mechanoreceptors) respond either to light touching of hands or to the grip of a strong handshake. Others concern themselves with the on/off of the touch (the onset and the release of the handshake) or the continued deep pressure of touch (a long, strong handshake does this). Touch receptors give us valuable information about vibration, the position of our body parts - such as an extended hand - in space (proprioception), texture, and temperature (Thomas

---

[152] Field 2001

and Reise have particularly warm hands; mine are consistently cool). Were I to painfully squeeze the hand I'm shaking (for the sake of theory here - I'd never be so mean in real life!), signals of pain would be sent from my client's hand to their spinal cord, where a reflexive pulling back would be initiated, even before the pain actually registered in their brain. Also, given that the palms of our hands have no hair (glabrous skin), certain receptors unique to these types of skin would activate, while the hairy (non-glabrous) skin of our fingers would signal another form of touch, the "caress" touch.

This touch, the "caress" as neuroscientists have named it, is a pleasant sensation and there are dedicated nerves that connect their nerve endings in the skin to the brain. These, amongst other nerves bringing touch information to the brain, come together in a place we've seen before: the insula. Here sensory events of many modalities converge, with the goal of deciding what emotional and hormonal responses are the most relevant and adaptive. However, we neuroscientists don't yet understand how we respond differently to a mechanical touch (being tapped on the arm by a pen) and an interpersonal touch (someone tapping your arm with their hand). Nor do we know how the tactile is integrated with other senses.

When I touch my client's hand in our handshake, I'm activating areas in their brains that process touch (somatosensory cortex) and the movement of our hands and forearms are covered by areas (motor cortex) next to the sensory cortex. The mapping of the areas is interesting: our body parts are represented along a strip of cortex, one strip in the front of the large central sulcus that separates the frontal and parietal lobes (primary motor cortex) and one behind this fissure (somatosensory cortex). We have head and neck and chest and legs, etc., all in a line. Interestingly, not all body parts are represented to the same extent: our lips and fingers are grossly distorted, with their maps covering relatively huge parts of the cortex, indicating their importance to our functioning and reflecting the higher number of neurons involved in servicing these areas. Some body parts are out of line, such as the genitals, which are positioned next to the toes (Foot fetish, anyone? Or having "cold feet"?). These are the primary sensory areas, responsible for receiving the initial information - *I'm in contact with something or someone* - from receptors in the skin; afterwards, the signals are sent to secondary or association areas, such as in the parietal and temporal lobes of the brain, to get more meaning (*I'm shaking* Erin's *hand.*). We use phrases and terms to highlight this role of touch: someone is "out of touch with reality" or they are being "tactless;" a movie is "touching" or our feelings are "hurt."

The right touch can have significant physiological repercussions, such as its ability to decrease stress (HPA flashback?) and lower blood pressure.[153] Interestingly, we encounter oxytocin (remember that "cuddle" hormone?) released here, as touch is fundamental to our abilities to bond. I think of Glenn, for whom I "prescribed" oxytocin for

---

[153] Whitcher and Fisher 1979

nightmares and anxiety in Chapter 1; he reaches for a reassuring hand-squeeze multiple times per visit. Is he subconsciously doing so for a burst of much-needed oxytocin? It wouldn't last long, as oxytocin works at first contact, not sustained pressure. For that, Glenn's endogenous endorphins (our natural feel-good, calming opioids) would have to be recruited; the good news is that oxytocin can trigger a full cascade of endorphins.[154]

But what if you don't have even a weekly warm handshake? What if you have no close relationships involving interpersonal touch? The majority of our clients have no partner, no "best friend." Are they lacking in the "touch oxytocin"? It would leave them particularly vulnerable to adverse neural, behavioural, and immunological consequences of not having a "touch relationship." They would likely be lonely.[155]

However, if you were to give Thomas, Ulmer, or Reise oxytocin, many if not all of these symptoms could, according to some researchers,[156] resolve. In other words, oxytocin could buffer the body from the varied effects of loneliness. But ethically, should we be providing an easy spray of oxytocin or the admittedly more laborious, and potentially fickle, solution of getting people together socially? I wonder if, given the choice, which would my clients choose?

---

[154] see Dunbar 2008

[155] Between initial writing and final editing, the Covid-19 pandemic came upon us. The resulting loss of much of our interpersonal touch has yet to be determined. Having been on maternity leave since just before Covid-19 hit B.C., I'm not sure what will happen in terms of touching clients.

[156] Dunbar 2010

A happy spritz in the nose or messy-but-rewarding human relationships? Would the oxytocin wear thin after a while, lacking in the complexities of friendship to carry it along? After all, there is more to loneliness than needing a "cuddle hormone." There is the longing for the sharing of thoughts and feelings; for rituals - daily, weekly, yearly - to add depth, and a shared trove of memories. The intricacies of emotional, social, and spiritual bonds with another person are far more complex than that of only one of the neurochemicals involved (i.e., oxytocin, endorphins). Do we therefore choose friends for our clients, playing match-maker, pairing up those we think might get along? How much of that role do we take on ourselves? Are we our clients' friends, in a loose sense of the word? "I look forward to this all week," Thomas noted regarding our Thursday visit.

Alone ≠ Lonely; Lonely ≠ Alone

These are pertinent and crucial questions, given that there is an increased likelihood of disease (morbidity) and even death (mortality) among people, such as Thomas and Ulmer, who have told me that they, living alone, are often lonely.[157] Being alone does not necessarily mean feeling lonely, though in some of my clients' cases, yes, many of them disclose as not just alone, but lonely. Loneliness, being a mismatch between the amount of social contact you want and that which you actually receive,[158] is a significant emotional distress syndrome, considered by some to

---

[157] Cacioppo et al. 2015
[158] ibid.

be a true, pathological, disease.[159]

They say it bluntly: loneliness kills.[160] The poorer mental and physical health of the lonely can deteriorate to the point of suicidality, as well as putting the lonely at higher risk of various physical ailments. This "hidden killer" is considered by these researchers to be "more dangerous than smoking." This is all the more problematic, and somehow ironic, given that many people, such as Thomas and Ulmer, both smoke regularly and report loneliness. I wonder if smoking works to relieve feelings such as loneliness, though they don't articulate this link.

My clients are typical in that loneliness presents itself disproportionally in older adults: Ulmer is among the 32% of people over 55 years of age who assert being lonely, while Thomas fits in with the 20% of those over 65 years of age who report significant loneliness.[161] As the general population ages, we will see more and more elderly people reporting feeling lonely. But loneliness affects other ages as well. The Canadian city of Vancouver, British Columbia (where I live and work), while being a relatively "young" population, is known as a "lonely city." People in their 20's to early 40's have difficulty meeting potential partners here, despite our numerous secondary institutions, bars, and other places to typically meet a mate. Many turn to dating websites. (Me, I simply met a new neighbour while we were doing our respective weekly laundry in our building's common laundry room... and we, twelve

---

[159] Tiwari et al. 2013
[160] ibid.
[161] Masi et al. 2011

years later, have been married over five years. You just never know where a chance encounter could happen! But perhaps we are an exception?)

Spitting image of cortisol

Loneliness directly and negatively impacts our immune, neuroendocrine, and cardiovascular systems. We've seen the neuroendocrine HPA axis before and its role in stress, and it is applicable here also, in the context of social stress. Were we to test the saliva of our clients who self-report chronic loneliness, such as Thomas or Ulmer, we would likely find higher levels of cortisol, suggestive of a malfunctioning HPA axis.[162] The actual levels would vary according to the time of day, though it is interesting to note that both of these clients are "morning people" and wake early. Upon rising, they, as people who report being lonely, would likely have more cortisol in their spit than other people (everyone has more cortisol in their system soon after waking; in the case of loneliness, the levels are particularly high). Cortisol levels in the saliva correlate with the loneliness of the moment, and also with the loneliness of the day overall.[163]

Immunologically, people living with loneliness are at a disadvantage.[164] Cortisol, that HPA axis output, can restrict glucocorticoid activity, which then provokes inflammation. This inflammation can result in diabetes, hardening of the arteries (atherosclerosis),

---

[162] Cacioppo et al. 2015
[163] Doane and Adam 2010
[164] Hawkley and Cacioppo 2010

and tumour metastasis - and even the death of neurons (neurodegeneration). Our levels of cortisol are predicted by the previous day's stress, and loneliness predicts the levels of cortisol even better than other stressors.[165] All this "just" from loneliness!

Another axis involved in our experiences of loneliness is the SAM (sympathetic adrenomedullary) axis. This system involves the inner parts of our adrenal glands (the adrenal medulla), which release norepinephrine and the well-known messenger, adrenaline (a.k.a. epinephrine). Recall that norepinephrine and adrenaline mobilize the body's systems to GO. This can happen quickly, which is great if there is an imminent threat that you need to deal with; chronic activation, however, is detrimental to one's health. At the level of the neuron, its receiving ends (synapses on its dendrites) may fail to grow, or the neuron may initiate its neuronal programmed death sequence (apoptosis).

Norepinephrine release is regulated by the PFC, and limbic regions (e.g., the amygdala and hippocampus) - that is, by our executive PFC and emotional limbic system. In turn, the amygdala, with the BNST (bed nucleus of the stria terminalis, if you must know), tells us about our stress: the amygdala likes to tell us of the stress that is happening *right now!* while the BNST tells us about the stress after it has started, but that goes on, and on, and on... often even after the stressor has gone away. Both are relevant: sometimes loneliness is acute, while other times it remains chronic. If, for example, Ulmer feels

---

[165] Cacioppo et al. 2015

that his "wife" Isabella is arriving imminently he may feel pangs of loneliness his amygdala sends out, while when he is thinking he has to wait a few years for their reunion, that loneliness is drawn out (BNST?) and less sharply felt. Personally, as I write, my husband is out of the country for a month. The first few days, I missed him terribly, and felt very lonely for him. As the weeks passed, my loneliness was sort of a dull ache, present but not upsetting. Now he is due home in a few days, and my loneliness has once again become a more intense, sharp feeling as I anticipate his return. That's the dance of my amygdala and my BNST.

Lonely homes

Housing can in part determine someone's level of loneliness, and just as one can be alone but not lonely, so also can one be surrounded by people yet feel intensely lonely. Many of my clients live in the single-room occupancy housing (SROs): large, old buildings - many built decades or even a century ago as hotels - that house as many residents as there are tiny rooms. (We don't mind a cramped hotel space for a week's trip away, but who would want to live entirely, day in and day out, in a twelve-by-twelve-foot room?) Some buildings are specialized for those with a mental illness, with staff there during the day to keep the peace.

Governmental funding has erected some newer buildings with slightly larger accommodations (including your own bathroom and kitchen area, thankfully). Many of these are built with those with mental health/addiction challenges in mind. They are staffed, have a meal or two included, and have a med program with nurses to administer. They've thought of everything. But does this make sense? Think about it: imagine you have developed, instead of schizophrenia, diabetes. Would you like to be told, "Oh, you have a disease. We're going to give you no option other than to live in a building filled with diabetic residents. It's for your own good: healthy meals, a medication program, a nurse on site! Oh, and since government funding only goes so far, you're going to have to live near the DTES."

Putting together 135 people with major mental health and/or addiction challenges in one building does not sound right (practically and ethically). Such a situation presented itself a couple of years ago: a new building housing that many residents. Should we be surprised when it becomes chaotic, a building we ACT staff must now go to in pairs, not alone, to safely see our clients there? And though the comings and goings of each tenant is observed by many residents, for many, there is little connection. Someone could easily live amongst the 134 other people while yet feeling cut off and alone. Voices and paranoia preoccupy many of our clients, further sealing them off from social connection. What resident will feel kindly towards a co-resident when their sleep has been thwarted by that neighbour spending the entire night screaming at their Voices... again? At times these neighbouring tenants will speak to us ACT workers when we are knocking on the client's door: "Can't you tell them to stop yelling all the time?" they demand angrily, and with good reason. Screaming at Voices is not uncommon for our clients, and this

185

greatly disturbs other residents. We sometimes fear for their safety because of it.

The older SRO rooms are tiny, and the bathrooms are communal, located at the ends of the hallways. Once upon a time, the hotels must have been grand and new, clean, and suitable for a few nights' stay. Now, rodents run around while many tenants hoard garbage (bringing cockroaches) and dirty clothing (harbouring bedbugs). Often the rooms smell, though the hotels' hallways and stairwells might be swept or mopped. Carlin keeps his room tidy and clean, but he still gets the mice and bugs that his neighbours' messes sustain. Miguel's room is his workshop, tools scattered everywhere and electrical or mechanical projects laying here and there. Reise has been binning lately, and his suite has piles of clothing to be worn again or sold, as well as a table full of cigarette butts that he repurposes into those hand-rolled cigarettes. Most have drug paraphernalia lying around, and we bring new sharps containers as needed to avoid the hazard of uncapped used rigs.

And the rent? About $400, give or take, for all of the above. This is generally paid directly, before the remainder of the government-issued PWD (Persons With Disability) cheques are sent out, lest it get used otherwise and the recipient be found without money to keep these "homes" over their heads. The government conveniently puts those living in such sub-standard SRO housing in their "housed" tally, making it look like fewer people are homeless. Much of Vancouver's population probably has no idea of the real living situations of the poor and marginalized; I didn't, not before joining ACT. The housing crisis for this population is severe enough, without the government further equating SRO's with "housed." Ironically, it is not uncommon for a person to choose to be homeless rather than live in an SRO hotel, especially during Vancouver's warmer seasons. It is not fair.

Each hotel has a multitude of suites (each being small), but despite plenty of co-resident contact, many people are isolated in the sense that they have few, if any, close trust-based relationships with their neighbours. Carlin is paranoid that others are forcing their way into his suite, and Miguel also believes this about his room. This keeps them suspicious towards other tenants, not friendly. I seldom see my clients socializing with other residents, though Miguel, the exception, has found a best friend a few doors down.

When others make us lonely

Not all of my clients live in such places. Glenn, for example, lives in a lovely, clean, and quiet complex. He maintains his small bachelor suite well and has a cat. Being mental health housing, there is support staff on site. Glenn often gets lonely, though, and wants to be able to go to staff with his problems, victories, and daily happenings. This, he reports to me weekly, distresses him. "The staff are so rude to me! I just tell them something, and they don't care. I hate living here!" he cries, wanting desperately to move out of this environment. "They play favourites, you know. Tracy goes to them and they give her so much attention. Then when I go, it's like: 'Glenn, you have the ACT team and your sister. Tracy only has me.' Why are they so mean to me? I'm never talking to them again. I'll just stay in my room and never go out!" But he does go, again, and again, always with the same results. He may have us at ACT and a positively involved older sister who helps him in many ways, but when he wants to share some tidbit from his life, he goes to the people at hand: staff. The rudest response Glenn has gotten is: "What am I supposed to do - clap for every little thing you do?"

Glenn has a similar relationship with one of the other residents of the complex, Tracy (the same Tracy as mentioned above). Glenn seeks her out, or accepts her arrivals at his door. He seems to have a pro/con relationship with Tracy: he recounts going to the store with her (pro) where she embarrasses Glenn by talking freely to strangers (con); he gives her things such as food he has changed his mind about eating (pro) but then she tells staff, contributing to the negativity Glenn sees from them (con); Tracy promises to repay him when she borrows money (pro) which Glenn regrets when she doesn't follow through (con).

I think loneliness drives him to expect great things from both staff and Tracy. He vows he is a "loner, like my Dad was" and that he wants to stay, insulated, in his suite. Yet, every week, he is complaining about staff's and/or Tracy's behaviour towards him, when he went to one of them. Loneliness does lead to a hyper-vigilance for social threats; for Glenn, this causes him to be biased towards attending to the negative in social interactions. Any inkling of rejection by staff will leave Glenn with an intense confirmation that exacerbates the slight. His PFC, a place of executive decisions, is to blame for that, while his hippocampus fails to link positive memories with social interactions. His surveillance for social threats is likely related to activity in his insula and ACC[166] and to his history of traumatic mistreatment.

As loneliness increasingly becomes seen as a disease, interventions can be developed. These include the pharmacological (oxytocin?) and the social. The latter would involve changing Glenn's social cognition: how he processes interpersonal interactions, and what he thinks are the reasons these people do things "to" him. Intervention at this level, that of social cognition, is thought to be the most effective, beating out medication. In CBT or other similar programs, Glenn could learn how to deal with his irrational beliefs (*staff should always drop everything and attend to me*) and false attributions (*if staff can't fulfill my needs, they don't like me*). In other words, faulty social hypotheses need to be examined and challenged.

Today, though, Glenn, his sister, and I met with a BC Housing assessor. The consensus - from Glenn's feelings, his sister's opinion and also my take - is that Glenn is ready to graduate from this tier of housing services. He has proven that he can do for himself many of the tasks the building is designed to do for their tenants: Glenn manages his own medications, cooks his own meals, and keeps his suite tidy and clean. He responsibly looks after his beloved cat. All this in combination with his personal issues with staff suggest that Glenn is ready for housing that

---

[166] Cacioppo et al. 2015

has fewer supports. There is a wait list for his current housing, as it could be used for someone who needs it more than Glenn does. The assessor agrees: it is time for Glenn to "move on."

Glenn is thrilled. He can't wait, but it could take the system many months to find a vacancy in another building for him. There is no specific timeline. If today is any indication, this wait will be hard for him. His anxiety today was difficult to manage, even though the stressor - news about moving - was a positive for Glenn. He took two prn clonazepam tablets and also went to the bathroom with a nervous bladder five times over the hour while we waited for the assessor to arrive. I know Glenn well, and foresee more anxiety as he waits. His limbic system is primed for intense emotions, particularly negative ones (amygdala territory) while his hippocampus dredges up memories of his past, perhaps ones in which he had lost out on something he really wanted. New memories (today's assessment meeting, for example) and old emotions of anxiety will likely mingle, as he is prone to thinking that if he has to wait, something bad must be going to happen. He has difficulty using his PFC's executive powers to keep these emotions in check, but with strong and frequent reassurance, his distress will diminish.

Lonely people groups

Increasing social contact is another way to treat loneliness. Glenn draws this from his twice-weekly visits from ACT, but resists other social engagements. ACT staff Yvonne has been encouraging Glenn to try out the one group that could mean the most to him: a supportive group of transgender members. Glenn has, over the past few years, transitioned, from female to male. He binds his chest as he waits on a long waitlist for "top surgery" (bilateral removal of the breasts) and wears men's clothes. I have had the honour of assisting him through the paperwork of legally changing his name, the sex designation on his birth certificate, and various other formalities. He looks, walks, sits, and even wears his excess weight as a man does.

Glenn unsurprisingly "passes," which makes him very sensitive concerning which bathroom to use when we are at the mall. "Sir, you're in the wrong bathroom," he has heard when in the women's restroom; he has fears around using the men's room. Thankfully, there is a "family" one that he feels most comfortable in. I support whatever his decision of the day is, reminding him that the choice to make is his. In sum, Glenn is, in my mind and his, male. He feels alone in this, sometimes asking ACT staff, "Am I a freak?" Yvonne has therefore been consistent and persistent in encouraging Glenn to try attending a group meeting of trasngender people. Yvonne has offered to go with him, and, given her people-oriented personality, she would bridge well between Glenn and other members of the group until he could do so on his own. I think this would do great things for his self-esteem, loneliness, and, by extension, his anxiety.

Generally, ACT promotes social contact for our clients, evidenced by our weekly DBT (dialectical behavioural therapy) group on Mondays - "Monday Wellness Group - and CBT (cognitive behavioural therapy) group on Thursdays. These types of therapy have been suggested as effective for loneliness.[167] Also offered by ACT are a smattering of other programs that bring clients together in a social setting, such as art group, exercise group, summer camping trips, picnics when the weather is warm, and activities such as bowling. Here, also, clients can pick up on social strategies and focus less on negative social stimuli. For a while, the Thursday CBT group was called "Miguel's Coffee Group," after my client, Miguel, and his uncanny ability to interact with every possible attendee in a positive manner. In doing so, he contributed to their social cognition: he is both an example of social aptitude and a non-threatening way for others to practice their own developing social skills with him.

As much good as ACT groups do for our clients, there could be the criticism that it is always, well, with *clients*. There are many positives for getting people with similar problems and/or life situations together, such as feeling understood and empathized with, but it also retains an insulation from society. Is it reinforcing the "client" identity, and a subtle message that *you are not ready for, or worthy of, contact with "regular" people*? That's how I felt in the groups I attended as a client. I wish our society were such that people with mental health and addiction challenges were embraced by community group activities. There they would feel included and taught skills in an as-needed, naturalistic way from members of their communities, as peers. While I idealistically dream of

---

[167] Cacioppo et al. 2015

such acceptance and inclusion, I do remember the many intra- as well as inter-personal skills clients have learned from client-focused groups. Moreover, I think that ACT's efforts to take a subset of our clients on camping trips in the summer is brilliant for establishing peer links among the participating clients.

Voices against loneliness?

I wonder: could there possibly be any link between hearing Voices and loneliness? I know that when I was little - I recall the third grade in particular - I spent many a recess at elementary school "playing" with my Voices. They liked the game "Stop/Go" where I would run at their "Go!" and become abruptly still at their "Stop!" This is the very game other children enjoyed, though they, of course, played it with each other. Carlin reports the same, and we agree that the Voices were kind then, when we were children, not the harsh, criticizing ones we hear now. For others, at times, their Voices still might give them something to smile about, some joke or slight. Many times I have seen a smile spread across Ulmer or Rachelle's face as they responded to an amusing inner Voice. Might these Voices provide some relief from feeling lonely? But then, Ulmer has been reporting having a "listening device" put in his ear, which sends his Voice-hearing into full drive; at the same time, he has noted more loneliness. So simply hearing another Voice does not necessarily mean that it will provide any relief from loneliness. In fact, Voices may make you even more lonely. They can taunt you: *what a loser... you have no friends...*

everyone hates you. They can also make you feel even more alone because no one "gets" you or believes you about your Voices. Stigma is pervasive and contributes to the feeling of loneliness.

The presumed excess of dopamine activity in the brains of people with schizophrenia may make us crave social contact even more than other people do; disturbed oxytocin levels may be key in our lack of social engagement, too. In fact, these changes in the functioning of dopamine and oxytocin, which influence each other in the amygdala, relate to deficits in social cognition in schizophrenia.[168] Maybe that's why we sometimes identify with our Voices; even their derogatory litanies may be better than no contact at all. But despite our suffering, when the Voices are unusually quiet, we, as Carlin and I have discussed, then feel oppressed by their silence. The private nature of our Voices makes them a further barrier to engaging with others, and as such might be both cause and effect of loneliness among people with schizophrenia.

We also exchange stories of the times the Voices amuse or help us. Carlin laughed when I told him that my Voices were imitating my colleagues' voices. Carlin, in turn, values his Voices' predictions of professional athletic game outcomes, on which Carlin places small bets in a lottery-type system (SportsAction). I am sworn to secrecy about the exact methods the Voices use to pick, but I can say that the Voices are sometimes quite right. I suspect Carlin's solid sports knowledge and experience - he was a

---

[168] Rosenfeld, Lieberman, and Jarskog 2010

rising hockey star in his teens - has something to do with his accuracy. I point out that he's giving the Voices credit when the real mastermind is his own intelligence! To that he smiles, and has, later, noted the same: "They're taking my credit away." (I admittedly love it when a client of mine begins to assert something I've been telling them for a while, when they *own* it... but then they credit themselves with the insight! Ah, my ego wishes they'd properly attribute that to me. But no matter - they are growing, and whatever the reason they acknowledge, I do rejoice.)

Loneliness and spirituality

Loneliness prompts us to look either inside to our own resources or outside ourselves for some support. Some people turn to the comforts of religion or spirituality. Communities of those who share spiritual beliefs often offer friendship and belonging, as well as inspiring purpose and hope. However, very few of our clients are attached to such a community, despite citing loneliness as a major hurdle in their lives. Religious institutions fund and staff a variety of charitable activities in the DTES, from homeless shelters such as the Union Gospel Mission to sandwiches distributed from the back of a van by my friend's church at a DTES park. The recipients need such physical interventions, but their spiritual needs must also be met if they are to overcome their loneliness. Such spirituality - or lack thereof - is as varied as the number of clients I meet with each week.

Chapter 9

God, or Not: Schizophrenia and Spirituality

"I'm with Einstein," declared Thomas. Not something I heard everyday working on the ACT team. But then, Thomas's background is hardly typical for an ACT client: he has a BSc in Physics and Mathematics. This intelligent man, now in his 70's, was answering my question, "Do you believe in God?"

"Einstein said, 'God doesn't play dice.' That's what I believe about it. That there's God," Thomas said.

This quote, one of Einstein's more famous ones, is thought to relate to the mysteries of quantum mechanics - the very subject that Thomas was most intrigued by in physics. But Einstein had focused his work on clear, definite theories and formulae (how much more elegant could his $E=mc^2$ be?). How could he reconcile this with quantum mechanics, where all seems to be random chance? That statistics - such as the probability of any roll of the dice - are our best estimate of how things operate at the most fundamental level?

Was Einstein meaning to say he was theistic, or at least deistic? This has been fiercely debated, with some declaring him a firm believer in God, while others certain he was an atheist. Thomas seemed to side with the former. He takes it to mean that the "dice" God does not "roll" corresponds to a fundamental purpose to everything, including we biological beings. It is like God doesn't take chances with His universe, and has a say in every force and in all matter by a fundamental organization of nature. It seems that Thomas is neglecting the quantum mechanics he leans towards.

I don't correct him. I don't really care if he is misinterpreting Einstein or not, because the quote gives Thomas a religion of sorts. It gives him a belief that all that has happened to him in his life has a non-random meaning. In his view, God has not abandoned him in a world of chaos, but has a non-chance meaning for us. God, in not rolling the dice on Thomas, would make him wanted, not a statistical accident. And that is a sentiment I want Thomas to have, especially as he ages and becomes, with each passing month, older. I worry about his physical health; he has voiced more than once that he knows he is in the "dying half of life." When I asked him to participate in this book, and mentioned interviews, he asked for the questions ahead of time, to prepare thought-out answers for me. He also stated wanting me to get to the interview quickly, before his answers were "blank... if I die."

While Thomas comes across as a believer in an

ordered universe, propped up deistically by a God, Miguel embraces a theistic faith outright. Although Miguel doesn't mention it often, when a good thing has happened - or when multiple, difficult "bad" things happen - he does make reference to "the love of Jesus Christ in my heart." He thus identifies with a traditional Christian creed. But he doesn't just believe in Jesus Christ as his own "saviour;" he holds to the belief that he is himself an angel from God. At times, on a certain level, I tend to agree with him; I chose his pseudonym in this book - Miguel - because it means "who is like the Lord." Miguel has this uncanny ability to put anyone at ease with witty, familiar conversation - people from any walk of life, be it a homeless person out collecting bottles for change, a fellow ACT client, myself, or even Wynn, a high-ranking officer of the Vancouver Police department whom he knows and respects. (You may have recognized Wynn's name from earlier in the book, as the one who helped me get my job at ACT. Wynn, Miguel, and I meet up for coffee every few months or so.) Expertly, but without an unnecessary polish and pretense of his expertise, Miguel brings a smile to another's face; he tends to pose and answer real questions instead of the superficial chit-chat that too often dominates conversations. This natural intelligence and gift does seem to bring an other-worldly feel to the table, and I can't quite believe it isn't, in some sense of the notion, angelic.

Miguel is poor, as would befit an angel, but he is provided for, abundantly, by his own efforts binning - and "luck from Someone," he states. He finds "armloads of stuff" every trip, and is equally generous with others, distributing his finds. Miguel embodies the opposite of selfishness. Things flow into his home, and out to his friends (and sometimes his enemies), as if he were a channel. Then, he goes out and there are again "armloads." I have often quoted the biblical to Miguel: "Give and it will be given to you. A good measure, pressed down, shaken together, and running over." (Luke 6:38) It seemed to fit.

Of note, Miguel has had a multitude of misfortunes, losing all his worldly possessions time and time again. He has no family to speak of, and many of his would-be friends just use him, discard him for the things of his they want. He has been homeless many times, only to be slotted into an SRO in between. He has been abused, neglected, hurt, and deceived. And yet, not a study in bitterness, only a thanks to "Jesus Christ in my heart."

Then there's Glenn, who is fiercely atheist. He cites God's lack of care for him in letting him suffer the way he did on the psychiatric hospital wards. He strongly feels that, "If there is a God, I hate him. He didn't hear me or help me." Glenn's anger is understandable, given those atrocious experiences in the hospital. "They left me there, naked, in the room, and locked me in, laughing at me," he tells me. They spoke meanly to him, belittling his suffering, both psychiatric and personal. Now he suffers PTSD-like nightmares of being in the hospital and only manages physical-health related appointments at hospitals with much emotional support. Where, he asks, is a loving God? Nor does Reise believe in a good God, but curses a God who brought him into this life. He is at times bitter, at times angry, at what he has received as his lot in this life. He's unsure of God's existence.

Spirituality is often pursued among a community of fellow believers, yet neither Reise nor Miguel nor Thomas attend a church; no rituals are performed. Even definitions of spirituality, such as an "orientation towards transcendent reality... a personal search for connection with a larger sacredness"[169] doesn't always capture my clients' outlooks on life. For many of them, day-to-day stressors - substandard housing, drug addiction, mental illness, and poverty - keep them focused on the survival of the here-and-now. The theological musings of a spiritual realm, either as a place to be in an afterlife or a balm for the present, doesn't always help them. The "central tenet"[170] may be "connection to something greater than oneself... finding meaning that relates life and the universe" but this search has for some been hijacked by drug use. After all, heroin may be described as a "big, warm hug" from a seemingly transcendent, omnibenevolent Being.

Aaron stands out from this crowd. His spirituality is clear and vibrant. He, being of Indigenous ancestry, finds great comfort, strength, purpose, and fulfillment in knowing his Creator and the creation of people and places He has made. About a year ago, I was honoured to have been the ACT worker to bring Aaron to the centre at which he chose to undergo intensive, residential substance use treatment last summer (one based on the values and

---

169 Van Cappellen et al. 2016
170 Mohandas 2008

practices of Indigenous cultures); I was even more honoured and humbled when Aaron invited me to pick him up, and to witness his graduation ceremony. I had always seen a glowing spark in Aaron, and now it came bursting out as Aaron left his heroin use behind him. Because the centre was based on Indigenous spirituality, Aaron found strength and hope in its practices. On return to Vancouver, Aaron tried out many supports, such as AA and NA (narcotics anonymous) groups, but felt the most support and growth in Indigenous practices such as his Talking Circle, daily prayer and smudging, sweat lodges, and Wellbriety (Indigenous cultural awareness in a 12-step recovery program). His awe at the transformative power of having his spirit name bestowed on him is pure and deep. Having a certainty about the goodness of his Creator has brought much goodness to Aaron's life and the lives he then touches in turn. For this first year or so of his recovery, Aaron has focused on himself and the spiritual work he needs; soon, he will "help others" find similar peace and purpose. It is always a joy to spend time with Aaron (and he has a perfect sense of humour to boot!). Interestingly, as Aaron no longer depends on an antipsychotic (his psychosis seems in hindsight to have been drug-induced) he may be a living example of the research that has found that increased spirituality is associated with decreased need for psychiatric treatment.[171]

My place is decidedly with the neurotheologists: scientists who study the intersection

---

[171] Grover et al. 2014

of neuroscience and theology. (Thomas accurately tagged me as agnostic.) Believing that our brains are sufficient to biochemically hold any of the millions of ways to be spiritual actually excites me, awes me, humbles me - states usually associated with spirituality. The reduction of spirituality to synapses and neurochemicals is not entirely helpful; we must not lose sight of the psychological and social aspects of religious belief. But my strong inclination is that our synapse-full brains not only underlie spirituality, they are actually and ultimately able to give us any of the variety of spiritual experiences humankind has found.

Oxytocin again?

Some research has implicated oxytocin in spirituality. Remember oxytocin, the "bonding" hormone important for the mother-infant bond, couples' trust (it figures prominently in orgasm to that end), and "in-group" loyalty? Well, oxytocin also figures prominently in neurotheology. This is not surprising, given that "spiritual" emotions such as comfort, peace, and trust are important in prayer, meditation, and other religious rituals, and these are the very emotions oxytocin mediates; stress reduction is clearly in the bag of tricks of oxytocin.[172] Oxytocin increases the salience of spiritual beliefs and produces the altruism and empathy central to many religions and spiritualities while decreasing the focus on oneself and redirecting it outwards to others.[173] One

---

[172] Holbrook et al. 2015
[173] van Cappellen et al. 2016

group of researchers[174] said it well: oxytocin leads us to "tend and befriend."

First, then, let's look at two correlational studies. In one,[175] 34 university students were asked to self-report: "To what extent do you consider yourself a spiritual person?" Their levels of endogenous (natural) oxytocin were measured by a simple saliva test, which is thought to be a quite reliable way of measuring oxytocin levels. These two bits of data were assessed for correlation. They fit! The more spiritual a person rated themselves, the more oxytocin they had going through their system. Interestingly, that correlation that held for spirituality did not appear when they tried to correlate oxytocin with religiosity ("How frequently do you attend church activities?"), just as Miguel and Thomas see themselves as spiritual without religiosity. However, I must note that the students in this study all attended a religious university (Brigham Young University in Utah - the central hub of Mormonism) and only one person rated their spirituality as less than 5 or 6 out of 7 (7 being the highest)… though, I noted, this one person also had the lowest level of oxytocin. These results could not be explained by mood, optimism, sex, or relationship status. In another correlational study,[176] endogenous oxytocin levels were twice as high in the participants who had reported a "spiritual transformation." These participants, men living with HIV/AIDS, may be unrepresentative of the general population, but the correlation between oxytocin and

---

[174] Kelsh et al. 2013

[175] Holbrook et al. 2015

[176] Kelsh et al. 2013

spirituality stands.

Mere correlation is not causation, but it is a start, and it can be interesting. It is, however, not surprising that another group of researchers decided to go beyond correlation and do an actual experiment looking at the relationship between spirituality and oxytocin. In a double-blind study,[177] researchers administered oxytocin or a placebo via a nasal spray to 83 men (a study involving women is in the works). 40 minutes later, the men were asked, "Right now, would you say spirituality is important in your life?" They replied using: importance = 0, 1, 2, 3, or 4 (a "Likert Scale"). They were then guided through a 20 minute meditation; the participants had reported not having meditated before. Their emotions were assessed using an adapted test involving spontaneous ratings of such emotional or spiritual words as "awe," "hope," "inspiration," "guilt," "sadness," and "anger." One week later, their spirituality was re-examined.

The participants couldn't guess with any accuracy whether they received the placebo or the oxytocin. However, the assessments found a clear relationship: oxytocin boosts spirituality more than a placebo does, both immediately and even a week later. The oxytocin-dosed men felt more interconnected with others, derived more meaning from their lives, and felt a greater sense of purpose. (This was independent of their emotional states.) Interestingly, the effect of oxytocin was stronger for those who reported no religious affiliation. This all

---

[177] Van Cappellen et al. 2016

suggests that oxytocin alone can *cause* a deeper, more meaningful spirituality. I wonder if a related molecule, vasopressin, can be called up here, too. Vasopressin and oxytocin work together to promote feelings of social connection and unity.[178]

Other neurotransmitters involved in spirituality include dopamine (levels go up), serotonin (also up), glutamate (likewise) and endogenous opioids (up again); cortisol, epinephrine, norepinephrine, and GABA levels all go down.[179] It makes obvious sense, if we recall the "stress" axis (HPA axis, that is) from earlier chapters which works with cortisol and norepinephrine as messengers of states of stress. Interestingly, the GABA, which normally makes the "thinking" parts of the brain (i.e., the cerebral cortex) calm down, here works (in the thalamus) to stop thinking "separateness" and begin feeling a connection to the outer environment. We feel "as one" with others and with our God. GABA might do this by fiddling with the sensations of our placement in space (proprioception), leading to our feeling less like separate human beings and more like the ultimate conjoined twins, without self-associated physical boundaries.[180]

Back to the beginning...

What does this all suggest about our beliefs in a God (or many gods, as the case may be)? Since oxytocin is a bonding hormone, it makes sense to

---

[178] Yaden and Newberg 2016
[179] ibid.
[180] ibid.

envision a personal deity to whom one can be emotionally attached. A God provoked by oxytocin may be the ultimate pro-social being. That is, your God must be good ("prosocial") and powerful ("ultimate"). Prayer to such a deity may increase your levels of oxytocin, making you feel safe. Glenn, as we have seen, is no such believer, and he struggles to feel secure. Perhaps he is missing out on some oxytocin? Earlier I wrote about Glenn's nightmares and anxieties and the potential therapeutic role of oxytocin, and here I am wondering again about this hormone for him.

Many studies on spirituality and meditation have been done, and there is a long, at times inconsistent, list of brain regions that "light up" in fMRI or PET scans when spirituality is evoked in the participants. My interest piqued when I noticed that several studies cited the involvement of the PFC and the ACC, as well as a mention of the insula. Also interesting: spirituality can evoke a response equivalent to a placebo effect.[181]

Remember the ACC and insula from our discussion of the salience network? Well, this network could be implicated in spirituality as well; not surprisingly, given that attributions of meaningfulness are key to one's spirituality. The spirituality that is unique to our human species may be linked to our ability to put faith (*I believe in God*) and meaning (*my God has a plan for my life; there is a heavenly reward after this life*) together. A candidate for this role is that group of neurons we saw in Chapter 2:

---

[181] Kohls et al. 2011

our von Economo neurons (VENs). Recall that these specialized neurons look different from other neurons in the cortex (longer, well-myelinated axons; bushy dendrites). As we saw, they are only present in a small set of mammals: those with (presumably) complex inner lives such as ours.

But what do these structures do in us?

Beyond these structural implications, there are also the functional ones. EEG studies, which focus on the functional activity of the brain, are common, particularly due to the portability of EEG machines. They could be brought to remote areas for testing monastery-bound meditating monks, and so researchers have been doing this for more than 50 years (since 1957).[182] With this technology, these researchers have found that Tibetan monks, when meditating, have an overall slowing of their brain waves. They are not sleep-like, though; the participants instead tested as highly focused and attentive while, almost contradictorily, significantly relaxed.[183] Remember the "beta breaks" we take when we calm ourselves down from the hyper, excited beta waves, and move to less anxious alpha waves? (See Chapter 3 for a refresher, if you need it.) The meditating monks' brains spend much more time in alpha wave activity, either at rest or when they are in meditation, than novice meditators who may still be struggling with the busy beta waves. Then there are the "theta bursts," which correlate to feelings of

---

[182] Cahn and Police 2006
[183] Schjoedt 2009

peacefulness and bliss. Finally, gamma activity - that tuning in from musical chaos, that "ah ha!" moment, that synchrony of neural activity we saw earlier - appears in meditators when they achieve the (superficially contradictory) depersonalization and self-awareness of a good meditation.[184]

There are significant problems with EEG research, though. Some researchers use too few electrodes, and their placement varies considerably from person to person and study to study, though more current (pun intended!) studies are more standardized. Still, there are many uncontrolled variables in how the meditations are conducted, and it is difficult to get groups of subjects that are matched in meditation experience and susceptibility. There is great debate over whether meditation studies' results reflect the meditators' ongoing psychology ("trait") versus the moment of meditation ("state"). In other words, is it "me" or "my activity"? Also, researchers are aware that there is considerable self-selection for meditation studies: *I'd like to be in your meditation study! I'm interested in meditation. Pick me!* Even if the participants have never meditated before, some of them are simply more likely to "get" meditation. When the research is with novices, perhaps those who arrive with more alpha waves to begin with are the most likely to remain in the studies. Confounding this is the fact that our EEGs change as we age.[185] Finally, there are just so many ways to meditate, so standardized consistency across studies is sorely

---

[184] Cahn and Polich 2006
[185] Zappasodi 2015

lacking.

At ACT, we follow the general trend of the research and believe that meditation is a great way to teach our clients to relax and improve their self-awareness. So on Monday afternoons at ACT, several clients arrive for "Monday Wellness Group" (MWG, in which, to repeat myself, principles of DBT, dialectical behavioural therapy, are taught). They are offered a way by which their psychological needs may be met. Specifically, a significant part of this group is learning about, and practicing, mindfulness and simple meditation. They are novices compared to the meditating monks, but still get a significant relaxation and focus from the MWG mediations. One of the group leaders, a social worker on our team, Aimee, has been counselling Glenn, teaching him meditations to ground him when anxious during the day or awoken by nightmares. The hope is that his nightmares and daytime anxieties will ameliorate with these stress-reducing exercises.

In practiced experts and novice dabblers alike, mediation has been shown to cause the release of GABA,[186] that neurotransmitter that "votes against" (inhibits) the postsynaptic neuron's firing. As we saw earlier, this GABA (in the thalamus) tells the cortex, the thinking part of the brain, to *quiet down, please!* Specifically, one of the areas affected is the parietal lobe of the brain, which keeps track of your body's contours and their placement in space; inhibit here (with more GABA), and you will find a feeling of being calm and connected to the things and people

---

[186]   Mohandas 2008

around you. Other neurotransmitters - dopamine and its role in sensing reward (dopamine is as much as 65% higher during meditation![187]) and serotonin that regulates mood, including euphoria - are also involved.[188] Add to that oxytocin's warmth and closeness and you've got a brain telling you either that you are near a divine Being or that you are at One with the universe, your interpretation depending on your spiritual beliefs.

God in a hat?

I'm intrigued: what else could artificially elicit spiritual experiences? In the late 1990's,[189] Michael Persinger, a Canadian neuroscientist, built a helmet equipped with small magnets near the temporal lobes that soon earned the nickname "the God Helmet." According to Persinger, when the electrical current supplying the magnets was turned on, the weak magnetic field would give you a sense of the divine. But the magnetic field employed was very, very weak. Less than that of one of your refrigerator magnets (!) and about a millionth of the strength used in TMS (transcranial magnetic stimulation, if you recall from Chapter 3). Subjects reported transcendent experiences of a "sensed presence," out-of-body sensations, and paranormal abilities. Cool - you can turn "God" on with a flick of a switch. But unfortunately, Persinger's result proved impossible to duplicate by other researchers, who instead found

---

[187]   Kjaer 2002
[188]   Mohandas 2008
[189]   as described by Schjoedt 2009

that suggestibility, sensory deprivation (the subject was kept alone in a dark, silent room), and a placebo effect were likely flaws in the original studies. In fact, researchers have since found that even sham helmets, and helmets that were not turned on, could produce the same results as the God Helmet, again suggesting suggestibility. Only certain people would sign up for the God Helmet, too, and when it was tried on Dr. Richard Dawkins, a scientist renowned for his atheism, he said that it "pretty much felt as though I was in total darkness, with a helmet on my head, and pleasantly relaxed... slightly dizzy [and] quite strange."[190]

Like I said, the God Helmet's magnetic force is a millionth of the strength of the magnetic force applied in TMS - the treatment that often silences auditory hallucinations. Interestingly, TMS over the temporal lobes (same place as the God Helmet) causes feelings of transcendence, and can enhance meditation. Maybe the God Helmet is on the right path - just too weak?

The God molecule, then?

So, maybe not a God Helmet, but what about the "God molecule"? Otherwise known as DMT (dimethyltryptamine), this "God molecule" or "Spirit molecule" is an entheogen: a chemical that makes us feel an experience of "God." DMT is a psychedelic, in the same class as "magic mushrooms" (psilocybin being the active substance therein) and LSD (lysergic acid diethylamide a.k.a. "acid"). They are essentially a

---

[190] Bogdashina 2013 p. 176

short-cut to transcendent experiences. Meaningful, spiritual, and mystical effects are common and may last for years.

Neurologically, epileptic seizures in the temporal lobes of the brain, aptly termed "temporal lobe epilepsy" (TLE), can be associated with mystical or spiritual experiences. In fact, the ancient Greeks considered TLE as "the sacred disease"[191] because of this. While none of my clients have been diagnosed with TLE, my friends Yves and Ethan have. For Ethan, the diagnosis of TLE came after that of schizophrenia, and ended up eclipsing it: the label of schizophrenia was deemed secondary to that of the TLE. That is, Ethan's schizophrenia symptoms are fully explained by TLE and having the diagnosis of schizophrenia is superfluous; it has been dropped. Yves's case, however, is more complicated. Given a rare and extreme sensitivity to the anti-seizure medication he was trialled on, Yves does not take medication for his TLE. He does continue with his antipsychotic, olanzapine (without weight gain, you may recall). However, he endures countless TLE seizures, which for him manifest as déjà vu, mutism, and absenteeism. He can be in the midst of a conversation and suddenly be unable to talk for a period of time. We, his friends, know to wait it out, but it becomes awkward when Yves is in the middle of a presentation - a relatively common event, as Yves often speaks publicly about his experiences with schizophrenia and the mental health system to such groups as police officers, high school students, and

---

[191] Yaden and Newberg 2016

nursing students. Interestingly, the brains of people with TLE and experienced meditating monks show similar brain wave activity, and both groups often report profound spiritual feelings of detachment, unity, and joy. People with TLE are more likely to be hyper-religious, and find many ordinary experiences to be profoundly important.[192] So do people with schizophrenia, making the separation of TLE and schizophrenia even thornier on a behavioural level.

Coping

Then there is the intersection of spirituality and schizophrenia. People living with schizophrenia often identify as spiritual and/or religious. Researchers[193] are attempting to determine whether people with schizophrenia use religiosity as a positive or a negative coping tool. On the plus side, spirituality can give hope, purpose, and meaning; on the other hand, there can be guilt, fear, and despair. As reported in one study,[194] 71% of participants used spirituality in a positive manner, while for 14%, spirituality was detrimental to their mental health. In other words, spirituality often helped reduce their symptoms of schizophrenia, though it could also increase them. Similarly, spirituality affected substance use, social integration versus isolation (loneliness), and adherence to, and acceptance of, treatment for their schizophrenia.

Positive coping in the context of schizophrenia

---

[192] Mohandas 2008
[193] Mohr 2006
[194] ibid.

reflected such non-violent sentiments as "if you say that God is love, you try to learn to love people."[195] Belief in a God and an after-life can give a hope of a heavenly reward for earthly suffering due to a mental illness, poverty, and other unfair stresses. Voices, such as Ulmer's, may be believed to be the Voice of God, or of angels/spirits, which may comfort and give psychological strength. It is also common, however, for the Voices to be the devil or demons; in these cases, spiritual beliefs may provoke feelings of punishment or persecution and thus contribute to negative coping. Recall that Reise often expressed that he feels his birth was a curse, and Glenn believes that if there is a God, he is cruel. Miguel, however, finds purpose and meaning in his spirituality, despite set-backs and adversity. In all these lives of coping, it is hard, if not impossible, to disentangle schizophrenia from the spirituality.

Religious delusions are associated with increases in a variety of negative indices:[196] more meds and, despite this, more symptoms and a decreased quality of life; self-harm and violence towards others increase; and proliferation of "poor outcomes" occurs. On the other hand, many people with nascent schizophrenia may seek religion out: their first plea for help, in response to their encroaching mental illness. Or, it could be a first sign of decompensation for someone with schizophrenia. I think of Thomas, and his sudden, intense interest in Catholicism when his mental health was failing

---

[195] Mohr 2006 p.1954
[196] Grover et al. 2014

earlier this year. He landed in the psych ward after being found in a church; his home boasted a new Catholic cross, rosary, and a large, ornate Bible. He asked me to please bring these items to him in the hospital, but staff said that the cross could be used as a weapon (the irony was not lost on me!) and refused to allow it. I think Thomas later gave the Bible away, but the cross now hangs on his wall at home, beside a print of a painting of Christ. The offerings of "food" (scrapped vegetable peelings) and knowledge (i.e., a Physics textbook) are gone, now. Interestingly, when I asked Thomas about his religious leanings, he replied, "Catholic and Buddhist... because they're basically the same." I queried what the similarities could be, as I thought them so different. "Love," Thomas said without hesitation. "They're both about love." I can't argue with that tolerant and personally meaningful take on theology!

Thomas is thus likely one of the 45% to 80% of people living with schizophrenia who use religion and/or spirituality to cope,[197] perhaps to cope with the loneliness we examined in the last chapter. Overall, the majority of our clients may interpret their symptoms and the related treatment through a lens of spirituality, and we ought to be aware of, and sensitive to it. Unfortunately, our team rarely discusses a client's spirituality and when we do, it seems that it is almost always considered in the negative light of psychopathology. For example, when Thomas waxed religious we certified him to the psych ward. We assumed it was his grandiosity and

---

[197]   Grover et al. 2014

psychosis, and it was indeed so. But it was also giving him comfort in a stressful time of emerging psychiatric symptoms. I wondered if Thomas's purchases were connected to his recurring comments, as a 71-year-old man, on feeling the eminence of his own death. Perhaps these feelings are a reconnection to the God and religion of his upbringing, to give him a sense of peace.

All this won't tell us whether or not a God, or gods, exist, only that human nature is such that there are biological, neurological, psychological, and social correlates; there are both benefits and drawbacks, of spirituality. Our well-being within ourselves and altruism towards others are clear benefits of spiritual engagement, in whatever form fits each one of us. Those benefits consist of longevity, improved physical health, decreased anxiety and depression, and reduced recourse to suicide.[198] These are interconnected, in that if, as a group, spiritualists are less likely to kill themselves and more likely to be in good physical health, then the average longevity of the group will increase. However sought, adding meaning to life is a good thing, one which we at ACT should be aware of and be able to help our clients hold onto. This is especially important when we consider the opioid epidemic in Vancouver, particularly in the DTES, where many of our clients reside, because lives are needlessly being lost to drug overdose. Miguel's list of friends and acquaintances who have died from overdose is long - 30? 50? He often wonders aloud why he has survived to age 62

---

[198] Mohandas 2008

(his birthday was a few days ago, so it figured prominently in our discussion this week). He has used drugs for about 50 years without major incident. In such times of mourning, spirituality can offer comfort, hope, and meaning. Miguel's tears remain, though; spirituality cannot bring the dead back to us in the here-and-now. But we can learn resilience from these life events. Indeed, could having the wherewithal to reach for spiritual aid be related to our being resilient enough to grasp meaning beyond our physical and social milieu? The answer to that question belongs in our next chapter.

Chapter 10

Resilient Rebuilding

"Everything. Gone. Again."

A small, very small, fire had given Miguel's landlord a wanted excuse to evict him, and Miguel had salvaged very few of his belongings. He was moved into a small, loud, and unsafe SRO with hardly anything in his possession. Angry, Miguel raged at the injustice of it all: the lame eviction excuse, the lack of follow-through from ACT in getting his stuff and the lack of housing options. And he was more than right to rage. It was far beyond unfair; some people had dropped the ball heavily but he was the one hurt.

Miguel has lost all his possessions several times before. He's been homeless. He's started from nothing several times in his life but he always picked up new things binning to replace the ones he'd lost. Because of this tendency of his, we at ACT floated around the term "resilient" to describe Miguel. Miguel was and is indeed highly resilient; he has an active and adaptive way of coping that creates opportunity and progress in his life, no matter what. He would rebuild. He always has, after all. One person, close to Miguel, suggested that this is simply a "reset."

I knew all of this, and did believe in Miguel's ability to have adversity not knock him down or out. He had done it for decades. I was, however, resistant to the term *resilient*. I did see and believe in Miguel's tendency to regroup, reassess, and resume his life. I did not, however, want to belittle what he had unfairly lost. *Oh, he's Miguel. He's resilient. He'll be okay.* Yes, Miguel would be *okay* but I think that attitude minimized his losses. "Resilient" should never be used dismissively, an excuse to trivialize. Those who, like Miguel, are resilient may be able to reset and rebuild, but their work, both physical and emotional, on this should never be overlooked. It is hard for Miguel, really hard. Moreover, the fact that he has "done it before" should make us *more* sensitive to his current crisis, not less. In fact, it means that Miguel has not only to deal with his recent losses, but also he must do something with the questions he asked me: "Why *me*? Why does it always happen to *me*? Why am *I* the one who loses everything over and over and over again?"

That *why me?* echoes in my mind, but from a different voice. "Why *me*? Why does it have to happen to *me*?" Glenn asks repeatedly. As you may recall, Glenn suffers from what is likely PTSD. Haunted by his nightmares, Glenn fears sleep and endures vivid daytime recollections of those horrible dreams. "I had to pull something in my wrists, and then it came out as fangs inside my wrists." "They put nettles in my hands and made me make a fist. It hurt like hell!" "I died. They killed me." Their continued presence fuels Glenn's intense fears of abandonment and re-hospitalization. As his treatment team, we often see his tears.

On the surface, then, Glenn may not seem all that resilient, given his fragile emotional states. But dig deeper, and you will see it. It's in his having come clean from crack cocaine, a feat he's upheld for close to nine years now. It's from his attention to his mental wellness, diligently taking his medications and keeping his appointments with us. It's clear, too, when he takes the bus without complaint to get to his monthly blood work, when he hates both the public transportation and the blood work with a vengeance. He is willing to grow and learn and change, if that's what he needs to do. I think that that exemplifies resilience. Without resilience, Glenn would be stuck in self-destructive patterns, not growing and bursting through them.

There is a commonly-used analogy to illustrate resilience. Imagine a glass jar. Inside that jar, there are marbles, each representing a negative event or trait in your life. You can drop marbles in - set-backs like Miguel's losses or adversities like Glenn's treatment in hospital - but if you try to reach in and take them out, you can't get past the narrow neck of the jar. Some other marbles inside may be genetic tendencies, such as those towards addiction; exposure to drug use may be an environmental marble. What, in this, is resilience? A filling jar threatens to overflow, into mental illness, perhaps, or destructive behaviours. It could mean the end of coping: suicidality. Inevitable?

No. While we cannot remove marbles, we can imagine placing a wide ring over the top rim of the jar. Now, the marbles are contained. They no longer spill out and overwhelm. Imagine another ring - a stable home, perhaps, or a good social network; it could be ACT's involvement. It might be a job or a pet; Glenn is very connected to his cat, Kitty. Another ring; another. You can cope with the marbles life throws in by orchestrating the addition of more rings. You are safer, protected: you have become *resilient*. It may be unfair the number of marbles life throws in, things out of our control such as how much the government is willing to spend on poverty reduction and the treatment of addictions. We can, however, take charge in our lives and add what rings we can. Miguel has done so, forming new friendships with his co-residents on his floor.

Trauma and resilience

I'd heard, somewhere, about a therapy called EMDR (eye-movement desensitization and reprocessing), and recognized it when my former case manager tried to start it with me. She had scooted her chair over, putting herself into my personal space, and held up one finger and started moving it from side to side right in front of my face. "Follow my finger with your eyes," she demanded. I was angry and felt violated, particularly because this was done without my consent and also because I knew its validity and efficacy were questionable. EMDR is based on the premise that this bilateral stimulation lightens the load of past traumas, bringing about psychological wellness. The originator of this unlikely treatment, Francine Shapiro,[199] had noticed that her clients moved their eyes back and forth involuntarily when disturbing thoughts arose; she also observed this in herself. Shapiro then assumed that this eye movement could alleviate anxiety, such as that of PTSD, if the involuntary eye movements were replaced with voluntary ones. I did not think highly of this idea at the time of my case manager's intrusion, and was not surprised at the dearth of scientific articles showing it to work.[200]

Then, however, I spent hours watching Miguel's eyes. Many of the 600-plus hours of the time we've had together (over five years of weekly, lengthy peer support visits) I have been looking Miguel in the eye. Most of that time, Miguel has been looking away, but he never seemed to mind my attentive gaze. From time to time, he would return the stare, perhaps to make a strong point or to look for understanding and validation. Interestingly, I have quite often observed in him EMDR-like eye movements: rapid, back-and-forth shifting. I knew from other cues, and from the content of his talk, that these moments were difficult ones for Miguel. Sometimes, with his eyes darting from side to side, he is silent - the kind of silence that invites no intervention from me. So I wait and watch attentively, letting him conduct his own, personal EMDR. I wouldn't base a scientific article on it, but it is interesting to note the similarities. At the very least, it kept me attentive to Miguel's emotional state and gave me reason to let him process his thoughts at his own pace. Perhaps it has served him

---

[199] Shapiro 2001
[200] Idler and Wagner 2006

well, his body's natural way of dealing with trauma. In any case, I'm not about to move my finger in his field of vision, nor do I care about the lack of well-designed studies on EMDR; I will focus on being present with Miguel.

Miguel generally leads where our sessions go; his loquaciousness (one of his favoured words) leaves few pauses. I don't speak much at the moment, but I sometimes want to relay to him what I'm understanding from our conversations. So I, a writer, write. Every so often, rather randomly, I draft a letter to Miguel about what I think he is trying to convey, both deliberately and unconsciously, during recent visits - particularly the deeper, underlying causes I'm seeing in him but that he has not quite articulated. I watch him read the letters; I am nervous. *What if I got it wrong?* I am acutely aware of my biases, misjudgments, and assumptions. But invariably, the response is, as he once put it: "You understand me at the nano level." I did pay close attention during those 600-plus hours. Every visit, I hear his words, as well as what he leaves out. I watch his facial expressions and those darting eyes. In my letters to Miguel, I detect, infer, and hypothesize. I quote him directly and also say what he seems, to me, to mean under many layers of difficult years.

A recurring theme is Miguel's self-worth. From our early days together, Miguel summed himself up as "an ignorant piece of shit." I reflected what I saw beneath that: *a golden core,* I said. We agreed on the fact that Miguel has done many negative things in his life, hurting others; we disagreed on his fundamental self-worth. Yet, years of visits and many positive letters later, I have not heard Miguel call himself that "ignorant piece of shit" for a while. In fact, he will list his strong points, almost asking *could this be true*? "I'm not bragging," he says to counter it, and I affirm that he is being accurate, not boastful. I see real, resilient change.

In turn, Miguel shares with me his poetry, new ones almost every week on a wide range of topics (the poems in the preface are authored by Miguel). These both - my outsider letters and the insider nature of his poem-writing - draw us closer together. Which is, we admit, strange, given the vast differences in our life experiences. But as Miguel said of it once: "We have fuck all in common... but you're my best friend." Something just works.

Suicidality I failed to hear

I have also failed Miguel, and he is in part resilient *despite* my work with him. I think of him now, and what he said to me last week. "You have failed me," he started. "All of you. ACT doesn't do shit for me. I told you my mental health was deteriorating and you guys did nothing. Nothing! You're not doing your job. It's pathetic. It's worse than nothing."

That's a lot to take in in ten seconds. My heart sank. *I have failed him.* Always before, Miguel had singled me out as the one doing things right, even while the rest of the team got his wrath. Since I am employed on ACT 2, and Miguel is a client from ACT 1 (Miguel and I were paired when the teams were just starting out, when they were a bit more fluid) I have less contact with the others who see Miguel and am often out of the loop. Miguel knows that when ACT surprises him with a *we're here to take you to an appointment/blood work/etc.* I have not known about it either. When, recently, Miguel was evicted from his home due to that small fire, he raged when one team member promised a second trip there to recover some of his belongings - but never followed up on his promise to Miguel. Later, another staff member told Miguel that "It only cost $500 to clean your place out!" which also hurt Miguel deeply.

Miguel was understandably angry with ACT, and detested his new "home" in the SRO. Weekly, I witnessed his anger and pain, and both he and I focused on his new accommodation as the source of his pain. He did tell me that his mental health was deteriorating, but I thought that he meant he needed to move, not medication. I listened to his anger, validated and normalized it, and reminded his team regularly that he needed better housing. I was wrong in this focus. In his recent assessment of ACT including me this time: I had failed him.

Yet, I was the one to whom he spoke more directly about it. Miguel had stopped by the office on a Monday, asking to see me, which was strange as our appointments are religiously on Tuesdays. "Here," he said, extending a pot of beautiful artificial flowers. "These are for you." I accepted them, and offered to go to the local park to talk. We sat on a bench and he was blunt: "At this point, I don't care if I die now. I know how I'll do it. It'll look like an overdose, but it's not." He caught my gaze and held it for a long, long time. His body posture was as if he had draped himself onto the bench, as if merging with it, as if he were dead.

"Are you considering suicide?" I asked, also blunt.

"Why not?"

We spent a bit longer there on that bench. I asked Miguel to walk me back to the office, which he usually does; he did. While he was in the bathroom, I had reception call down an ACT 1 staff member. "It's urgent," I pressed. Hattie came down, and I summed it up: "Miguel is suicidal and possibly psychotic," I said, and then Miguel appeared behind me.

"What's she doing here?"

"Miguel, this is too big for me. I'm worried about you."

Hattie took hold of the situation, and we talked outside. Miguel engaged, but when Hattie asked to speak to me inside, he figured it out.

"You're going to get the doctor, right?" he said angrily.

"Yes, Miguel. I'll be honest. You need to see a doctor." Hattie was clear.

"Fuck you!" Miguel hurled at us. "I don't need this shit." He stormed away.

Hattie, being a casual staff member, but the only one in the ACT 1 office at the time, called for a co-worker's opinion. They agreed on hospitalization, but - Miguel was not on Extended Leave. We could not "recall to hospital" (put him on the psych ward involuntarily). There was nothing to do; my witness had no authority, I was told more than once. The psychiatrist would see him the next day.

That evening was brutal for me. I really, really doubted I would see Miguel the next day, Tuesday, for a visit, either because of his anger at me and at ACT, or because... *What if?* I was nearly ill with worry this time. *What if...?* His team had plans to check in with him at the office, or otherwise go to his home at the SRO, to assess. Meanwhile, I worried. I wondered if the flowers had been a good-bye gift. Would Miguel follow through with his plans? This would prove to be my very worst day at ACT in all of my five-plus years.

But, Tuesday came and so did Miguel. I held back, and two members of his team met with him in the small conference room. At one point, I went down, and heard Miguel yelling at the psychiatrist. However, half an hour later, he was waiting for me and for a nurse from ACT 1. He was going back on a long-lasting injectable antipsychotic. He held still for Nicholette - "Do you want to see my bum?" he added, always one to add that touch of humour - and accepted the IM in his gluteal muscle.

That's what he wanted. Miguel was, as he has done in the past, using expression of suicidality to convey his need for help. I had thought the housing was the focus - that he was saying that he needed to move for his mental health. Obviously, I had missed his point. I did not recognize his desire for this kind of intervention. I had been thrown off that trail because he has in the past, abhorred and resisted psychiatric treatment. My heart ached: I had hurt him; also, I damaged our relationship. Ironically, up until that visit of blatant suggestion of suicide, I had thought that I was helping with just my empathetic listening and attempted housing advocacy. I was wrong.

Unjustly, staff on ACT 1, after checking in with Miguel on Tuesday, belittled my concerns from the day before. It seemed as if they thought I had overreacted. *Miguel wouldn't kill himself. Why did you make a mountain out of a molehill?* After all, he seemed more than fine on Tuesday. But, knowing Miguel as I do, he was truly suicidal on Monday. Perhaps I was able to pull through for him enough to turn him around. I don't think he wanted to die, but that he was feeling that there were no other doors out of his psychological pain. Such hopelessness, combined with ready means to kill himself (drug overdose) are key factors when assessing the risk of suicide. I think he was asking for my help, and I think I got the right help for him, finally.

The suicidal brain

Suicide is among the top ten causes of death in the world, and there are around ten million attempts each year. The definition of what constitutes a suicide includes lethality and intent, though these are at times unclear. When a client dies from a drug overdose, we simply cannot always know whether it was accidental or intentional. Either way, we grieve the loss of life.

As with any human experience, suicidality is associated with distinct neurobiology. Sadly, much of this knowledge has been obtained post-mortem, but it nevertheless promises to help those still alive but at risk, such as Miguel. He has become suicidal before, notably earlier on in our relationship: he used to express having thoughts of suicide whenever I took my vacation days, telling no one until he told me upon my return. This was a heavy burden on me that

I tried to share with his team. However, Miguel has never to my knowledge attempted suicide actively. Sometimes, he mentions a passive overdose of his dope as a possible outcome when he uses it, yet he remains resilient, mostly focusing on the positives in his life. What, in Miguel's brain, could correlate with this interplay between his resilience and an intermittent suicidality?

Here we encounter BDNF again. It is significantly decreased not only in those who die from suicide (no matter their psychiatric diagnosis) but also in those whose behaviours suggest suicidality.[201] In Chapter 5 we saw that BDNF is also critically low in schizophrenia, and this may relate to the high (10%) risk of completed suicide amongst those living with schizophrenia; I was myself nearly such a statistic. Developmentally - and schizophrenia is considered to be a neurodevelopmental disease Miguel's serotonin "happy" system may have been impacted by low levels of BDNF.[202] In the absence of BDNF, our NMDA receptors fail in ways that hinder neuroplasticity: that is, BDNF makes it harder for our suicide-sensitive brains to learn from, and adapt to, the trials of the environment around us.

And, adapt to the environment within our brains. As people who have considered suicide at our lowest points, Miguel and I may have disruptions in multiple neurotransmitter systems, such as those of serotonin, GABA, glutamate, norepinephrine... but not dopamine, interestingly (recall that dopamine

---

[201]   Paska, Zupanc, and Pregelj 2013
[202]   Sher 2011

dysfunction is thought to be the major cause of schizophrenia). Cortisol is high in the urine of those who commit suicide.[203] The adrenal glands are larger, as if they are working harder than usual. Stress-evoked hormones affect the PFC[204] where decisions regarding suicide may be made. However, we don't really know which came first: the HPA axis stress response or the suicidality. We have to remember that indices of stress in those who have died, or nearly died, at their own hand are skewed: it is stressful to orchestrate your own death. It goes round and round: stress predisposes us to suicidality, while suicidality is itself stressful. What it really comes down to, though, is my role as one who connects emotionally with those clients of mine that are at risk. I try to connect them to feeling heard and valued, and to connect them to further help as needed. I try to offer them a meaningful oasis of purpose and hope, the acceptance of which varies tremendously from client to client.

Miguel and I recently had coffee with Wynn, a high-ranking officer in the VPD who has personal links to both Miguel (through an ACT camping trip) and me (Wynn was instrumental in my application to do peer support work at ACT: "I will open doors for you."). Wynn was describing his passion for education, particularly for the young. "Our lives are basically determined by the time we're seven years old," he said to Miguel and me. Miguel clearly latched on to this, and began recalling his life at age

---

[203] Tormey, Carney, and FitzGerald 1999
[204] Mann 2003

seven. He could see the connections. The abuse and neglect he endured from a very young age had a strong, negative impact on young Miguel. Such early stressors, both as lived experiences and as brain-based changes (for we, while focused on neuroscience, must always bring it back to "living level"), burrowed into him and dug down deep into his psyche. BDNF levels relate to childhood trauma[205] and I wonder how Miguel's levels compare with others, both then and now.

Yet, here remains Miguel. At age 62, he wonders how - and why - he is still alive, when so many he has known have died around him. He has an obvious will to live and is endlessly resilient, beautifully neuroplastic. I do not think he will kill himself, despite the occasional words and demeanour. But, I do not take the risk of testing this hypothesis. Having learned a lesson from the last episode, I hope to hear him earlier and more clearly, and get him help, as needed, sooner rather than later.

The photo that made Miguel speechless

As I have noted before, over the past few months, I had taken some photos of my clients on my work phone. It was time to print them out. One of my favourites was that one I'd taken of Miguel. We had, as you may recall from Chapter 4, been sitting outside in the pleasant weather, on a bench. It was the day after Miguel turned 62, and while I looked at him as he spoke, I found he looked really *good*. I said so: "Miguel, you look really good today. Can I take a

---

[205] Sahu and Jacob 2016

picture of you?"

"Sure." A couple clicks, and I showed him the photo on the phone. His response was quick: "I look like a bum." I didn't think so, but we left it at that. What I saw in the photo was the sun shining on his hair, an angelic halo, and the play of a smile on his face and in his eyes.

A few weeks later, after I had gotten the prints made, Miguel and I sat on yet another park bench. I gave him a copy of his photo. He took it, carefully, and settled. "I need to look at this," Miguel said quietly, and the loquacious man had no words. For a long moment - several minutes, I think, though it seemed like hours - Miguel surveyed his likeness. This time, there would be no "bum" remarks. He held it up, brought it close; he smiled at it, nodded his head. Finally, a remark: "I look happy."

"You were."

"This is the best picture anyone's ever taken of me," he said quietly. "Thank you." I accepted the thanks. He put it carefully back in the envelope I'd had it in, slipped it into his pack. He did so with much care. I had given him something very valuable. Those moments, as he contemplated his photo, are among my favourites in my five-plus years at ACT.

Walking proof

Aaron has been working hard, actively demonstrating the meaning of physical resilience. He has never given up on himself, and nor have we at ACT; we believed in him when he had almost stopped believing in himself, and that has been a good part of the foundation he has built on. We saw

Aaron's transformation of spirit in Chapter 9. Here, I note Aaron's physical resilience. He has undergone numerous surgeries, a broken femur, renewed infections, and pain that requires Kadian (an opioid replacement therapy that Aaron, with his physician, is tapering slowly). After several hip surgeries and much physiotherapy, Aaron progressed from wheelchair to crutches. He has transitioned from crutches to walking poles, to walking unaided. His goal is to hike the local "Grouse Grind" which is a steep and challenging mountain hike that is well-known in Vancouver. Aaron has been physically preparing for this with much dedication, both in physio appointments and his general activities (walking, biking, going to the gym). Sometime in the spring next year is his goal. I have no doubt he will complete this "bucket list" item, a perfect example of his physical resilience.[206] Psychologically, this will put Aaron in the mindset of *I can accomplish my goals with resolve and hard work.* He is careful to listen to his body, pushing or pulling back according to its signals; he knows that pushing too hard will only set him back.

These examples of resilience impress on me the importance of my being, as a peer support worker, "all things to all people." What one client needs, another does not, and each client of mine expresses their varied needs to me in different ways. As their peer support worker, I attempt to hear, understand, empathize with, and give hope to them. It is a

---

[206] Indeed, Aaron met his Grouse Grind goal in the time between the writing and the editing of this manuscript… and he immediately made plans to do the hike again!

demanding job - one in which I at times excel, at other times, fail - but I embrace it fully. I do love the connections certain clients and I have made, and we have made many good memories. For me, peer support brings out my own personal resilience.

Chapter 11

How We Are Peers

I remember well my most meaningful moment as a peer support worker employed on the ACT team. Aaron and I were completing an application for the residential treatment facility he had chosen to attend for his addiction to heroin. We had just filled out a full page of his use of any of twenty possible drugs of abuse: Do you use this substance? When did you start? How often do you use it now? What route of administration do you usually use? I felt honoured by Aaron's honesty, and his trust that I was a safe person to be doing this with, as he told me about this history. *Hard liquor at ten... heroin by his 30's.* I could sense his depletion. One more question on the page: *Have you ever had an eating disorder*? "No," Aaron replied, and I wrote that down, then paused. Would this be taken the right way?

"That's what I struggled with," I offered. "And I see a lot of parallels with my eating disorder and substance use. There's the shame, and the secrecy. Lost relationships and so much time, money, and energy gone. And hating it, not wanting to do it, wanting to stop - even while doing it. Feeling hopeless and beyond help."

Aaron looked me in the eye. "So you understand my addiction. You get it." It was between statement and question.

"Yes, I think so. I do."

We sat there a moment, quiet. I felt a profound sense of *no judgment* between us, and I think Aaron felt it too. We - with tremendous differences in our pasts and in our circumstances at that time - had a connection as peers.

I didn't think I would have a more meaningful moment again; and, this one would not have happened without the one I described above with Aaron. To back up a bit, Aaron and I have met weekly for a peer-to-peer visit, both before he went to treatment (the one we had been applying for) and after. I had the privilege of bringing Aaron to the centre, by taxi, ferry, taxi. I have no vehicle - all my outreach is by public transit - but, I was the one on the team who wanted to take on the long day of travelling from Vancouver to Vancouver Island and back. Aaron, being on crutches, needed help with his bags. It was also nice for him to have company on this long journey.

As noted earlier in this book, a number of weeks later, Aaron invited me to attend the closing ceremonies at the centre, and to accompany him home. True to a promise I made to him, he had new housing to come home to, far from the DTES and in a building whose mandate was focused on recovery. Aaron thrives in his new, clean life, and we have built a deep peer friendship. I believe we share tremendous respect for each other, and inspire each other to live with care, good intention, and empathy. We end each visit with that handshake, eye contact, and good wishes (though Aaron is far from the loneliness that other clients live with).

So, Aaron texted me one morning, asking to see me that day, even though it was not our usual day. "I have a gift for you," he wrote. We planned to meet at the office at 12:30. As I met him in the waiting room at ACT, he had a great smile on his face and a reusable shopping bag around his neck (his creative way of carrying it, as he is on crutches). We went into the side room, and he presented me with the bag. I peered inside, and was amazed, awed, and humbled. A drum. "I want to thank you for all that you've done for me, for being such a good friend," Aaron said to me.

"But this - it's the one you made, isn't it? It's too much..." I trailed off. He had shown me photos of it on Monday, a beautiful work of both art and meaning. I lifted it out, carefully, reverently. Aaron explained the rituals of making and gifting this drum: Indigenous traditions blessing it with smudging, washing, and tobacco. I held in my hands countless generations of tradition and faith in the Creator. I was awed. Tears nearly overwhelmed me.

"When you make your first drum, it is for someone else. I knew right away that I was making it for you."

"Thank you," I said simply, with emotion. "I will treasure this for the rest of my life." It was a tremendous gift, one that leaves you with deep gratitude. "Can I give you a hug?"

We spoke for a few minutes, sharing connections with our words and eyes. Another profound sense of humble awe in the human spirit. I had known Aaron since the days when his spirit was all but crushed by heroin, when he lived in the most derelict of an SRO building. But then, as now, I always saw his spirit, the spirit that now shone brightly. Aaron is priceless, blessing so many in his path. He traces his new life back to when he received his spirit name; now, later, he lives up to that name. Strong Horse. Today, a gift from Strong Horse to Peace, which is what my Irish name means. Overwhelmingly deep and precious. He knew my gratitude, humbly accepted. We parted, with a laugh and a smile.

Philadelphia

Such emotions are not well captured by neuroscientists and our hypotheses, and some others would shout *heresy!* to the examination of what the brain is doing when one feels that way. But just as any emotion or belief is written in neural code, so there are neurobiological correlates of love. Here, I refer not to romantic love, but to the Greek *philadelphia*, meaning *brotherly love*. Just as *philadelphia* is based on mutual respect, trust, and care, so also Aaron and I base our relationship on these tenets.

Neurobiologically speaking, the feelings of love are rewarding and feel good. Oxytocin, as we've seen, is a clear candidate, as are serotonin and dopamine. These three neurotransmitters are thought to be involved in friendship's bonding (oxytocin), happiness (serotonin), and sense of reward (dopamine). A great combination for the experience of love, and it is one that is sadly lacking in some of my clients' lives who may, as we've seen, have become quite lonely. Aaron, in contrast, certainly tends a wide, varied, and meaningful support network of family, friends, and elders, one in which he gives and receives care and love. This richness replaces his heroin addiction; he is so well-connected to others, I see no return to his former life that was artificially "loved" by heroin. We have heard that heroin, at least at first, is like a "deep, warm hug." It is a substitute, and in addiction it devastates. Thankfully, so thankfully, Aaron has passed, with intention and much emotional work, from that bare existence on heroin to such a full, loving life now.

A mirror to empathy?

In other words, Aaron and I aspire to be rich in empathy. For this, we depend heavily on our so-called *mirror neurons*. These neuronal cells were first observed by researchers[207] in monkeys, but let's extrapolate to humans; there is now evidence to support that leap. Mirror neurons are active not just when you yourself perform an action (e.g., reaching for a treat) but also when you watch someone else do the same. Unsurprisingly, mirror neurons are found in motor areas (*I can copy what you do*), but they have also been discovered in the parietal cortex[208] where more complex, associative things happen to our basic

---

[207] Gallese and Goldman 1998
[208] Chong et al. 2008

sensory and motor inputs. Some mirror neurons respond only when the action is the exact same, while others have some flexibility: they don't just mirror robotically and inflexibly; they say, *That's kind of what I was getting at*. This lets us interact socially, when we contemplate and work towards a common goal.

Mirror neurons are not just about the action; they care about motive. It's as if they mentally repeat the action while noting the intentions they'd have if they were doing that action. The action matching is trying to literally *walk in someone else's shoes* and mirror neurons let us do so while acutely but subconsciously aware that: ... *hmm, shoes... I know how to walk in shoes... this other person has shoes, walks... I wonder if this is what it's like to walk in their shoes... Is this what they experience?* Similarly, mirror neurons are thought to underlie the ability to imitate facial expressions, as even newborns can: they reflexively mirror some facial expressions even when they are only hours old.[209] When I see a client smile, I smile too, and feel the feedback from that smile as: *I'm smiling and feel happy; he is smiling, so he must be feeling the same.*

Could all this suggest that mirror neurons be the neural underpinnings of empathy? One researcher has suggested that mirror neuron empathy is a part of us that accounts "for all different aspects of behaviour enabling us to establish a meaningful link between others and ourselves".[210] Empathy, the compassionate understanding of someone's feelings, is what peer

---

[209] Meltzoff and Moore 1977
[210] Gallese 2001 p.42-43

support is all about. Other members on the ACT team, while highly compassionate, cannot *know* what it's like to live with a mental illness, as peer support workers do. True, no one can ever empathize with every person's exact circumstances and past experiences, and I, compared to most of our ACT clients, have had a very different, privileged life. I do, however, draw alongside them in their frustration with symptoms, their intolerance of medication side effects, or their feelings of helplessness when certified to hospital. I can empathize with meeting these challenges at times with despair and helplessness, other times with the satisfaction of regaining mental wellness. I know how much someone helping you accomplish small goals can make you feel heard and validated. However, I cannot *know* what it's like to be very poor, addicted to street drugs, and/or "housed" in an SRO downtown. I feel my privilege acutely and ask for the humility to be quiet and listen when I cannot speak from experience. Somehow, sometimes, it works. As Miguel said, and as I quoted earlier: "We have fuck all in common, but you're my best friend."

Friend? Am I? I am involved with my clients' lives because I am paid to do so, not because we are friends. On the flip side, I've had clients say to me, "You don't really care. You're paid to do this."

True enough, almost. In response, I offer: "You're right - I am paid, and this is my job. I am paid to spend time with you, and I am paid to do so respectfully. I am paid to treat you with dignity and offer help. But I cannot be paid to care. That, I do from my own reserves."

I try not to take work home but sometimes it

does follow. I do care. From week to week, visit to visit, I think of my clients, their lives, and what might be going on for them. I worry, I hope, I wish good things on them. To some, that is enough to call it friendship, and I accept that designation. Others, who I think esteem me just as much, call me "my worker" which is technically more accurate. I have to watch boundaries, both mine and theirs, and I do set limits on what they can know about me, although these vary from client to client. Like Miguel, Aaron calls me "friend" and with him, I return the word. With Glenn or Reise, I do not. I can't quite articulate my reasons why, but I go with my professional and personal instincts. I seem to *know*. I hope my intuition is there to best support my clients, individually, and that it helps keep them well. However, there are times when even an empathetic peer support worker is at a loss, and I let the team know that they need more help than I can give.

Risk of elopement: the psych ward

"We'll recall him," said the psychiatrist. He, the psychiatrist, is relieved that he, the client, is certified under Extended Leave. That means that there is paperwork already in place such that Thomas can be taken to hospital and committed without the psychiatrist having to prove that at this time Thomas needs to be certified in the hospital. The shoo-in. Now to physically get him there, which is no easy feat. Thomas, like most of our clients, could resist. That's when our ACT VPD officer could arrive, with authority and handcuffs.

Luckily for all, this time, Thomas could be

reasoned with. One of our ACT staff, a nurse, Natalie, knows Thomas as well as I do, and he trusts her when she says that he needs to go to the hospital. She brought him to Emerg, where the waiting began. After an hour, I spelled her off and sat beside Thomas in the waiting room. I didn't think he'd run off (at 71, he's just not quick enough), but I brought reinforcements to distract and keep him there: I doled out chocolates and applesauce packets from my bag every half hour or so. Thomas's intense frugality would never have allowed me to buy him a pop from the vending machine, but he accepted the treats from my bag happily. He kept the packaging, intending on finding those lovely sweets in the store and buying them to enjoy, though I know he will never deem the prices low enough for his thriftiness. But in the moment, they worked, and we were eventually called into the treatment area.

Thomas was given a small room and told to change into hospital pajamas. I stepped out, returned. I was out of chocolates, and Thomas was getting grouchy - understandably so, given our three-hour wait. He expelled a curt word to staff, and I was pulled from the room. They knew him at this hospital - it was not his first admission here - and they wanted to put cuffs on his stretcher *just in case*. I knew their reasoning but recoiled reflexively; I too have spent many, many hours in restraints. I emphasized the other ways to deal with Thomas: "He's very rational. Explain why you want to do something, and he will probably comply. Let him do things his own way, when possible." I'm thinking of his careful keeping of rinsed, empty milk containers and chocolate

243

wrappers - little idiosyncrasies that are too often what is focused on by hospital staff. Bizarre? Perhaps. Harmful? No. But, alas, the cuffs, indeed, went on the bed, against Thomas's loud protests, and I cringed, near tears, as I stood outside the door to Thomas's room. Traumatic flashbacks to when I was the one in the room with the cuffs.

Security left, and I composed myself and went in. Thomas was sitting on the bed, and I asked, "Can I sit with you?"

He looked at me. "Yes." I sat quietly beside him. We spoke, a little, about the cuffs. I let him know that I could empathize, and he received my words of comfort. But I couldn't stay forever, and I left Thomas alone in that room as I went back to the office, wrote up the required case note, and walked sadly home. I feared for Thomas; feisty as he is, I wondered if this hospitalization would be the death of him. Twice that evening, he had said to me, "You know why people go to the hospital? To die." I found out the next day that Thomas was put into restraints. Mad and kicking, he was transferred to a room in the new mental health building, where he would spend the next number of weeks.

Twice a week, I went over to see Thomas, bringing treats (more chocolates). But he was fading away, aging right before my eyes. His "contrariness" (his will) only got him seclusion, restraints, and forced injections. They gave him Haldol - an old, powerful antipsychotic - four times a day to keep him easy to manage. His gait became a shortened shuffle, his voice grew hoarse and strained, and he had neither the sparkle in his eye nor a smile. Rules on every side made him speak of killing staff in revenge. This worried staff: "Should we refer to tertiary?" By every account, in their view, he was deteriorating. Natalie and I agreed, though: it was the hospitalization that was, ironically, responsible, and we pushed for discharge. From this stance, the best word I had for what Thomas was going through was *demoralization*. Tertiary treatment - an extended stay - could well have killed him, spirit first, then body. After too many weeks of the psych ward, Thomas returned home. The next Thursday, when I bussed over to his place, Thomas opened the door with a smile and life in his eyes again. He had survived, without lingering or intrusive signs of trauma.

For Glenn, though, surviving psychiatric hospitalization was highly traumatic, and he has joined the ranks of the number of patients who develop signs of PTSD after repeated and stressful hospitalization. The use of coercive measures, such as the restraint, seclusion, and forced injections that Thomas, Glenn, and Miguel (and I) have experienced, can be indeed traumatic. The acute helplessness and fear is palpable.

Why would Thomas and Glenn respond to their respective experiences of hospitalization in such dramatically different ways? For one, Thomas's emotions were directed outward, at others, while Glenn took it inward, which may have made the difference in their outcomes. Thomas blamed the "rules" and snubbed them, while Glenn worried incessantly about being abandoned if he somehow broke the rules. Thomas vowed to hurt - even kill - others; Glenn hurt himself, if you may recall, by cutting, and by swallowing small but dangerous items such as batteries. In common was their dislike of hospital to the point of being a "danger to themselves or others." Happily, both Thomas and Glenn are home and well now; both are on clozapine.

Drowning in psychosis

With medication adherence, many of my clients, such as Thomas and Glenn (as well as myself) have found a certain peace. We may only take our meds because they keep us out of hospital, but we take them (you'd think I'd have more insight than that, but sometimes, it's the only thing making me keep taking my antipsychotics). Often this dedication comes about only after so many different trial-and-errors of type and dose and combination. My sweet spot is loxapine at night and Abilify in the mornings. These imperfect but effective drugs ground us.

A favourite analogy of mine for this is that involving a swimming pool:

Imagine that you are in the deep end, and cannot swim. You thrash and claw at the water, all your effort and stamina and hopes battling the inevitable drowning. If only you could catch just one breath! But one will not suffice; you need a series, unending; you are dying in the deep water.

That battle for life is the war we fight against schizophrenia. We drown in symptoms, desperate but growing weaker, succumbing. We will die.

But then - a table! Just like the ones we, at six years old, stood upon in after-school swim classes, that were tall enough to raise our heads above the waters; a table of medication had saved us from the deadly waters of psychosis.

For me, I had thought my schizophrenia had me; suicide was attempted. But then, my feet stumbled, fumbled as I stepped up on the table. Solidly there, I gasped and breathed good air in, out, in.

That medication is under me, solid; others are going through the long trial-and-error of finding that foundation. I, and at times my clients, stand, permitted now to rejoin the ranks of the breathers. We call out, for help; we are still deep in the waters. We may sing. We can embrace psychological resolution; we have space to begin talking to the psychiatrist (and, perhaps, a peer support worker). Friends and family may welcome us, no matter our being dripping wet and chlorinated. I have found the psychological support, but only because I was given a foundation of medication. It provided the stability for psychosocial rehabilitation, my recovery. I wish that for my clients, too.

Maybe, at some future point, I could learn how to swim. For some percentage of people with schizophrenia, there is possible remission. We are as yet unsure who and why these lucky few are, but we are at least now questioning the long-held belief that schizophrenia is necessarily life-long. Some residual symptoms may linger, but by definition, these are mild and do not interfere with the person's day-to-day and long-term functioning. Perhaps there is no cure, but there is, at least for some, *recovery*.

Ah yes, recovery. I will stick my neck out on this one: I do not like this term. Literally, it means to look backwards in time and take back what once was ours. But I can't "recover" past states; I have aged and grown and matured, and I will never be, feel, or think as I once did. Some things may be similar now as then, but never exactly the same. For example, I could, in theory, "recover" my high-school weight, but my body shape and fat and muscle distribution has changed, so even if the scale were to report the same number, it still would not have been "recovered." Were I to recover from schizophrenia, I would not hear Voices or believe rats were eating my brain, but having experienced those things has changed me to be more on alert, more cautious. My brain has changed, ir*recover*ably. I propose we do away with the term recovery and choose a new word: *dis*covery.

Discovery looks forward, not back, and says: *This is what I have right now to work with. Let me discover what I can do with this to make my future a better place.* Discovery is creative and strength-based. It does not limit us or tell me what should be, but rather what could be. There is hope, not bitterness; possibility, not a closed box confining one's potential. It may be on meds or off them; what matters is what gives us our quality of life. Recently, I shared this perspective with Aaron, and he absorbed it immediately. *My discovery,* he said.

My discovery: thinking about thinking

To help my own discovery, I have been participating in an extensive, detailed study of the effects of cognitive remediation treatment and metacognitive training. I have always had a love of

248

cognitive stimulation; I relax at the end of the day with a strategy game that keeps my mind active... I write books. I assume that steps taken to improve the mind could assist in the remission of cognitive challenges, or at least a better quality of life.

The cognitive remediation ("remediation" meaning to reverse/stop damage) I'm doing is based on a prescribed set of computer games, each designed to hone an aspect of cognition. This "Happy Neuron" program we use has become quite popular; they reference a number of clinical studies that support this program. However, there is a fee (after a seven-day free trial). People with schizophrenia are one of their target populations, one in which cognitive remediation has been shown to work, particularly when combined with other psychiatric rehabilitation.[211] Each Happy Neuron exercise focuses on an underlying skill - processing speed, problem solving, spatial memory, and attention, to name a few - that is supposed to generalize to daily living tasks. They are quite fun, though I admittedly am fond of cognitive challenges and did "max out" on level ten for all but one game. It's nice that there are no "side effects" of this treatment other than occasional frustration.

In metacognitive training we see a lot of hand-drawn pictures of objects and situations that we have to perceive, understand, and judge. For example, we are shown a couple of lines, then a few more lines added, then more, until the entire picture is outlined. We have to guess at each stage what the picture is; at

---

[211] see Wykes et al. 2011 for a meta-analysis

first, we have no ideas, but it becomes progressively easier to identify. Other times we are shown a cartoon block and have to predict what will happen. These sessions are group-based, and you probably get more out of it if you participate than if you just sit there. I try to be an active member of this group, in part to help keep it flowing along. However, I didn't want to be the only participant, so I at times hold my tongue and wait for others to say something.

As a part of these programs, I travel by bus to and arrive, always early, to UBC's Detwiller Pavilion for the MRI component. The maze we follow from the waiting room to the MRI suite brings back flashes of memories. I've wandered the halls of this building often, as a student, an inpatient, a staff researcher, and as a volunteer. I was keen on presenting my brain for the good of science, though not altogether altruistically (they paid me in cash, after each session. I've contributed the sum of $325 of data to science so far in this study). But the prize I take home today is a CD of my brain. 3D, I've been told. I'm not quite sure what the CD holds, but I fear this round, flat disk.

I know too much. I've examined countless brain scan photos; would I recognize the pathology? There would be the ventricles, the brain's reservoirs of its nourishing liquid (CSF, or cerebrospinal spinal fluid)... in schizophrenia, these spaces expand. "Enlarged ventricles" is the term researchers use. In this ventricular expansion, the fluid pressures change and disturbs fragile brain tissues. There, along the fault line of the ventricles, the insula thins. In people with schizophrenia, it has lost some of its grey matter although neuroscientists have yet to find out whether this pathology is brain development gone awry or a loss relating to the onset and persistence of schizophrenia. Given my history of problems with ascribing salience normally, I fear seeing my insula's thinness. Finally, I do not want to see signs of the general cortical "shrinkage" that has been reported for people with schizophrenia.[212] That is, my whole brain may be markedly, pathologically, irreversibly shrunk. Do I really want to see that? Will curiosity win over fear?

The ills of psychiatry; the ills of anti-psychiatry

As I contemplate my possible, physical brain deterioration, I feel pessimistic. If the very structure of my brain has changed significantly, such that my difficulties are not just an imbalance of neurochemicals but are an actual loss of brain, is there hope of true "recovery"? I am intrigued that while many researchers are finding those physical abnormalities associated with schizophrenia, others[213] are reporting that developing schizophrenia is no longer thought to predict a life sentence. Instead, remission can and does happen for some. Not long ago, remission from schizophrenia was seen as an original misdiagnosis. But for me? For my clients? Dare we dream of full mental health without our handfuls of pills every day?

There are diametrically opposed thoughts on this. In my lifetime experience of psychiatrists, the

---

[212] see Krause and Pogarell 2017 for a review
[213] see Zipursky, Reilly, and Murray 2013 for a review

vast majority of them will not wean you off your meds; they operate in fear of my decompensation. True, I've relapsed a multitude of times. Why would now be any different? The other side has also gone to the extreme. Instead of caution, they promote blanket mistrust of the entire psychiatric process. I will get to this topic in a moment; first, I have to introduce you to Evan.

Last week, I was with Evan, one of my newer clients. We are still finding our footing as we visit, but we both see it as a promising start. Recently, Evan had requested a review panel as part of his rights under BC's Mental Health Act. In his review panel, a group of people, professionals and others - including Evan and his advocate - would weigh in on whether Evan needs to be detained under Extended Leave (that is, involuntary treatment). A voluntary client can refuse medication and visits; an involuntary client cannot. We hold the threat of recall to hospitals over our involuntary clients, at times with a coercion that makes me cringe: *if you refuse your IM injection, we will recall you to hospital.* Evan, who felt that this force was not helpful in his life, had wanted the review panel. He was confident in his case, believing he would be freed from involuntary treatment with ACT. However, he showed his satisfaction with our new peer relationship by asking me, "If I get off ACT in my review panel, can I still see you?" I saw that as a good sign.

He didn't "win" the review (what horrible language we use for this). He wasn't overly upset, though, and did still want to see me. At one of our latest visits, he came prepared with one question:

"What do you think of the Mental Health Act?"

I responded openly and truthfully. Evan had been reading my memoir, so he had some idea of what I'd been through. "First," I said. "I without doubt would not be here, were I not treated for my schizophrenia under the Mental Health Act. I would have long since managed to kill myself."

Evan nodded. He had read the first chapter of my memoir, a serious suicide attempt in response to my Voices.

"That said, I am certain that I received much more involuntary 'treatment' than I should have. The restraints, the isolation in the 'quiet rooms', and the injections, forced on me when I was in my psychosis of utterly believing that the medication had those microscopic rats that would proceed to eat my brain. It was terrifying and I think it made things worse."

Evan could agree.

We talked further, noting the feelings brought up by the involuntary treatment we'd both endured. Evan had been kept on Extended Leave by his review panel; I'd been on Extended Leave a couple of times. We agreed on one thing: it makes you feel powerless. Apathy or anger could grow in such conditions, though neither Evan nor I have reacted with either of these extremes.

For the next visit two weeks later, Evan brought a topic of discussion again. He placed a magazine-like publication on the table between us. It was clearly about the evils of psychiatry and its pharmaceuticals. Evan wanted my opinion again.

I began to sift through the content of the magazine, finding both science I agreed with and alarmist conclusions I believed were unfounded. Evan watched me, but said little. It was the beginning of an intense visit.

The first topic I encountered was that our current antipsychotics have undesirable side-effects. "Without doubt," I said. "In 75 years, we will look back on the antipsychotics we use now and exclaim how problematic they actually were. After all, 75 years ago, you or I might've had a frontal lobotomy or an induced coma - 'treatments' we now see, rightly, as barbaric and ineffective. But that doesn't mean our current drugs aren't able to help some of us."

"But the side effects? They sound so dangerous."

"Definitely - the drugs do have side effects and these range from benign to severe. But keep in mind that when they list side effects they include every possible one, even if they only happened to one person. They do it not as science but to get out of legal repercussions. They're basically 'covering their ass' so they don't get sued."

"Huh."

"And, pharmaceutical companies indeed *are*, as I'm reading here, concerned with financial gain," I said, pointing to the next page. "There is more money in treating a disease than curing it. So they develop antipsychotics. But - and this is important - just because someone's profiting from us taking our drugs doesn't mean the medicines are not useful. Yes, they're getting rich off our drugs, but the reason they're selling is because they work."

"I never thought of it that way," Evan replied.

I flipped pages, reading quickly and

commenting on small points. Diagnosis of schizophrenia: "We can't physically peer into the brain and see the schizophrenia," Evan noted wisely. "We can't see chemical imbalances."

"No, we can't, not directly. A lot of research is with rats or mice, and they can't get schizophrenia the way people do."

Evan laughed at this. I smiled, too.

"But, we can infer some things with confidence," I continued. "A neurotransmitter can be broken down to other forms, known as metabolites. We then can measure how much of that metabolite shows up in blood tests, or in testing the brain's fluid by a lumbar puncture."

I paused, recalling in my mind that, indeed, many neuroscientists look at metabolites of either our endogenous neurotransmitters or of the drugs they give us. For example, dopamine is broken down to its metabolite, HVA (homovanillic acid). We measure this because dopamine itself does not cross the blood-brain barrier - but HVA does. HVA levels have something meaningful to say about the amount of dopamine being used in the brain (though not all the HVA in your circulation comes from brain dopamine activity). HVA levels are related to some symptoms of schizophrenia[214] and can predict how well you would respond to certain antipsychotics.[215] The worse your psychosis, the more HVA you likely have in your CSF,[216] indicating more dopamine at work in your brain.

---

[214] Veselinovic et al. 2018
[215] Mazure et al. 1991
[216] Maas 1997

I resumed my speech: "Some 'brain scans' help too. They can show if an area of the brain is bigger or smaller than normal. I know that a consistent finding in schizophrenia research is that our spaces for the fluid that nourishes the brain are bigger. Others - you may have heard of a functional MRI?" - he had - "can measure the activity of parts of the brain indirectly by seeing how much more the blood flows there. We're confident in these methods - just not always 100% sure of the implications of any of these brain abnormalities. Something can look bad on a scan but the person may have adapted and shows no signs of it in their daily life."

"Right... I see," Evan said, nodding his head. I could sense that he was about ready to end the visit. I'd talked a lot, and noted this to Evan. "It was good," he acknowledged.

"Would you like to plan another visit? I've given you a lot to think through."

"Yes, definitely. Our usual - in two weeks?"

"Sure." We left Subway and walked down to where Evan turned to cross the street, almost home, while I headed in the opposite direction to catch a bus back to the office. I hoped I'd helped Evan see both sides of the issues he had raised by bringing the publication, as well as how the magazine seemed overly alarmist and one-sided while still getting some things right. It will be interesting to see what he brings to our future visits. His intelligence and desire to hear different perspectives was clear that day, and our peer support relationship seemed off to a good start.

It's been good, having a new client. Evan and I

are "getting to know" each other and it is a rewarding phase.[217] Other clients (that I see regularly) and I have spent five years or more together. Miguel and I, as I already noted, have well over 600 hours of time together. It's never boring, though; people are endlessly interesting and I continue to discover new talents (Ulmer knows sign language!) and quirks (Thomas prefers bossa nova music). Challenges arise, are dealt with, and recede, whether they are mundane (getting new dentures for Glenn) or life-changing (finding housing for Aaron after treatment). Nothing is static. My clients teach me many things about life and I count myself extraordinarily lucky for their acceptance of me in their lives. *Through me despite me* is my mantra for every visit: *through me* means that, for whatever reason, I am the one interacting with this client at this visit and I can be the support they need; *despite me* reminds me that I will never support a client perfectly. My limitations are inevitable and I will at times say or do the wrong thing. This idea keeps me humble and opens me to whatever life lessons my clients and I will encounter, together.

---

[217] Sadly, after the writing of this chapter, Evan died.

References

Ahmed, A. O., Mantini, A. M., Fridberg, D. J., & Buckley, P. F. (2015). Brain-derived neurotrophic factor (BDNF) and neurocognitive deficits in people with schizophrenia: A meta-analysis. *Psychiatry Research, 226*(1), 1-13.

Angelucci, F., Brenè, S., & Mathé, A. A. (2005). BDNF in schizophrenia, depression and corresponding animal models. *Molecular Psychiatry, 10*(4), 345-352.

Araya, A. V., Orellana, X., & Espinoza, J. (2008). Evaluation of the effect of caloric restriction on serum BDNF in overweight and obese subjects: preliminary evidences. *Endocrine, 33*(3), 300-304.

Barak, N., Beck, Y., & Albeck, J. H. (2016). Betahistine decreases olanzapine-induced weight gain and somnolence in humans. *Journal of Psychopharmacology, 30*(3), 237-241.

Barr, R. S., Culhane, M. A., Jubelt, L. E., Mufti, R. S., Dyer, M. A., Weiss, A. P., Deckersbach, T., et al. (2007). The Effects of Transdermal Nicotine on Cognition in Nonsmokers with Schizophrenia and Nonpsychiatric Controls. *Neuropsychopharmacology, 33*(3), 480-490.

Barr, R. S., Culhane, M. A., Jubelt, L. E., Mufti, R. S., Dyer, M. A., Weiss, A. P., et al. Deckersbach, T. (2007). The Effects of Transdermal Nicotine on Cognition in Nonsmokers with Schizophrenia and Nonpsychiatric Controls. *Neuropsychopharmacology, 33*(3), 480-490.

Bartz, J. A., Zaki, J., Bolger, N., & Ochsner, K. N. (2011). Social effects of oxytocin in humans: context and person matter. *Trends in Cognitive Sciences*.

Bassett, K. E., Schunk, J. E., & Crouch, B. I. (1996). Cyclizine abuse by teenagers in Utah. *The American Journal of Emergency Medicine, 14*(5), 472-474.

Belfi, A. M., Koscik, T. R., & Tranel, D. (2015). Damage to the insula is associated with abnormal interpersonal trust. *Neuropsychologia, 71,* 165-172.

Berg, S. A., Sentir, A. M., Bell, R. L., Engleman, E. A., & Chambers, R. A. (2014). Nicotine effects in adolescence and adulthood on cognition and α4β2-nicotinic receptors in the neonatal ventral hippocampal lesion rat model of schizophrenia. *Psychopharmacology, 232*(10), 1681-1692.

Berna, F., Bennouna-Greene, M., Potheegadoo, J., Verry, P., Conway, M. A., & Danion, J. (2011). Impaired ability to give a meaning to personally significant events in patients with schizophrenia. *Consciousness and Cognition, 20*(3), 703-711.

Berna, F., Potheegadoo, J., Aouadi, I., Ricarte, J., Allé, M., Coutelle, R., Boyer, L., Cuervo-Lombard, C., & Danion, J. (2016). A Meta-Analysis of Autobiographical Memory Studies in Schizophrenia Spectrum Disorder. *Schizophrenia Bulletin, 42*(1), 56-66.

Berridge, K. C., & Robinson, T. E. (2016). Liking, wanting, and the incentive-sensitization theory of addiction. *American Psychologist, 71*(8), 670-679.

Berthier, M., Starkstein, S., & Leiguarda, R. (1988). Asymbolia for pain: A sensory-limbic disconnection syndrome. *Annals of Neurology, 24*(1), 41-49.

Bogerts, B. (1985). Basal Ganglia and Limbic System Pathology in Schizophrenia. *Archives of General Psychiatry, 42*(8), 784.

Boison, D. (2008). Adenosine as a neuromodulator in neurological diseases. *Current Opinion in Pharmacology, 8*(1), 2-7.

Boison, D., Singer, P., Shen, H., Feldon, J., & Yee, B. K. (2012). Adenosine hypothesis of schizophrenia – Opportunities for pharmacotherapy. *Neuropharmacology, 62*(3), 1527-1543.

Brashear, R. E., Kelly, M. T., & White, A. C. (1974, March). Elevated plasma histamine after heroin and morphine. *Journal of Laboratory Clinical Medicine.*

Brüne, M., Schöbel, A., Karau, R., Benali, A., Faustmann, P. M., Juckel, G., & Petrasch-Parwez, E. (2010). Von Economo neuron density in the anterior cingulate cortex is reduced in early onset schizophrenia. *Acta Neuropathologica, 119*(6), 771-778.

Cacioppo, S., Grippo, A. J., London, S., Goossens, L.,

& Cacioppo, J. T. (2015). Loneliness. *Perspectives on Psychological Science, 10*(2), 238-249.

Cahn, B. R., & Polich, J. (2013). Meditation states and traits: EEG, ERP, and neuroimaging studies. *Psychology of Consciousness: Theory, Research, and Practice, 1*(S), 48-96.

Cannon, M., Jones, P., & Murray, R. (2002). Obstetric complications and schizophrenia — a meta-analysis of population-based studies. *European Psychiatry, 17,* 10.

Carey, K. B., Maisto, S. A., Carey, M. P., Gordon, C. M., & Correia, C. J. (1999). Use of legal drugs by psychiatric outpatients: Benefits, costs, and change. *Cognitive and Behavioral Practice, 6*(1), 15-22.

Chong, T. T., Cunnington, R., Williams, M. A., Kanwisher, N., & Mattingley, J. B. (2008). fMRI Adaptation Reveals Mirror Neurons in Human Inferior Parietal Cortex. *Current Biology, 18*(20), 1576-1580.

Colton, C. W., & Manderscheid, R. W. (2006). Congruencies in increased mortality rates, years of potential life lost, and causes of death among mental health clients in eight states. *Preventing Chronic Disease, 3,* A42.

Conway, J. (2017). Nicotine and symptoms of schizophrenia: the 2017 picture. *Medical Research Archives, 5*(7), 1-11.

Corlett, P., Taylor, J., Wang, X., Fletcher, P., & Krystal, J. (2010). Toward a neurobiology of delusions. *Progress in Neurobiology, 92*(3), 345-369.

Covell, N. H., Weissman, E. M., & Essock, S. M. (2004). Weight Gain With Clozapine Compared to First Generation Antipsychotic Medications. *Schizophrenia Bulletin, 30*(2), 229-240.

Crespo-Facorro, B. (2000). S17.04 Insular cortex abnormalities in schizophrenia: Clinical correlates and significance. *European Psychiatry, 15*, s246.

Crump, C., Winkleby, M. A., Sundquist, K., & Sundquist, J. (2013). Comorbidities and Mortality in Persons With Schizophrenia: A Swedish National Cohort Study. *American Journal of Psychiatry, 170*(3), 324-333.

Daskalakis, N. P., McGill, M. A., Lehrner, A., & Yehuda, R. (2015). *Comprehensive Guide to Post-Traumatic Stress Disorder: Endocrine Aspects of PTSD: Hypothalamic-Pituitary-Adrenal (HPA) Axis and Beyond.* Switzerland: Springer International.

De Kloet, C., Vermetten, E., Geuze, E., Kavelaars, A., Heijnen, C., & Westenberg, H. (2006). Assessment of HPA-axis function in posttraumatic stress disorder: Pharmacological and non-pharmacological challenge tests, a review. Journal of Psychiatric Research, 40(6), 550-567.

De Kloet, E. R., & Oitzl, M. S. (2006). Cortisol and

PTSD: Animal Experiments and Clinical Perspectives. *PTSD*, 13-27.

De Kloet, C., Vermetten, E., Geuze, E., Kavelaars, A., Heijnen, C., & Westenberg, H. (2006). Assessment of HPA-axis function in posttraumatic stress disorder: Pharmacological and non-pharmacological challenge tests, a review. *Journal of Psychiatric Research, 40*(6), 550-567.
De Kloet, E. R., & Oitzl, M. S. (2006). Cortisol and PTSD: Animal Experiments and Clinical Perspectives. *PTSD*, 13-27.

Doane, L. D., & Adam, E. K. (2010). Loneliness and cortisol: Momentary, day-to-day, and trait associations. *Psychoneuroendocrinology, 35*(3), 430-441.

Dringenberg, H. C., De Souza-Silva, M. A., Schwarting, R. K., & Huston, J. P. (1998). Increased levels of extracellular dopamine in neostriatum and nucleus accumbens after histamine H1 receptor blockade. *Naunyn-Schmiedeberg's Archives of Pharmacology, 358*(4), 423-429.

Dunbar, R. (2010). The social role of touch in humans and primates: Behavioural function and neurobiological mechanisms. *Neuroscience & Biobehavioral Reviews, 34*(2), 260-268.

Dutton, D. G., & Aron, A. P. (1974). Some evidence for heightened sexual attraction under conditions of high anxiety. *Journal of Personality and Social Psychology, 30*(4), 510-517.

Ellenbroek, B. A. (2013). Histamine H3receptors, the complex interaction with dopamine and its implications for addiction. *British Journal of Pharmacology, 170*(1), 46-57.

Els, C., Kunyk, D., & Sidhu, H. (2011, June). Smoking cessation and neuropsychiatric adverse events. *Canadian Family Physician, 57*(6), 647-649.

Evins, A. E. (2000). Placebo-Controlled Trial of Glycine Added to Clozapine in Schizophrenia. *American Journal of Psychiatry, 157*(5), 826-828.

Field, T. (2001). *Touch.* Cambridge, MA: MIT Press.

Fox, G. B. (2004). Pharmacological Properties of ABT-239 [4-(2- -benzofuran-5-yl)benzonitrile]: II. Neurophysiological Characterization and Broad Preclinical Efficacy in Cognition and Schizophrenia of a Potent and Selective Histamine H3 Receptor Antagonist. *Journal of Pharmacology and Experimental Therapeutics, 313*(1), 176-190.

Freitas, C., Fregni, F., & Pascual-Leone, A. (2009). Meta-analysis of the effects of repetitive transcranial magnetic stimulation (rTMS) on negative and positive symptoms in schizophrenia. *Schizophrenia Research, 108*(1-3), 11-24.

Gallese, V. (1998). Mirror neurons and the simulation theory of mind-reading. *Trends in Cognitive Sciences, 2*(12), 493-501.

Gallese, V. (2001). The "shared manifold' hypothesis: From mirror neurons to empathy. *Journal of Consciousness Studies, 8*(5-7), 33-50.

Gaspar, P. (1989). Catecholamine innervation of the human cerebral-cortex as revealed by comparative immunohistochemistry of tyrosine-hydroxylase and dopamine-β-hydroxylase. *Journal of Comparative Neurology,* 279, 249–271.

Goodkind, M., Eickhoff, S. B., Oathes, D. J., Jiang, Y., Chang, A., Jones-Hagata, L. B., … Ortega, B. N. (2015). Identification of a Common Neurobiological Substrate for Mental Illness. *JAMA Psychiatry, 72*(4), 305.

Grover, S., Davuluri, T., & Chakrabarti, S. (2014). Religion, spirituality, and schizophrenia: A review. *Indian Journal of Psychological Medicine, 36*(2), 119.

Gurpegui, M., Aguilar, M. C., Martinez-Ortega, J. M., Diaz, F. J., & De Leon, J. (2004). Caffeine Intake in Outpatients With Schizophrenia. *Schizophrenia Bulletin, 30*(4), 935-945.

Hawkes, E. (2012). Making Meaning. *Schizophrenia Bulletin, 38*(6), 1109-1110.

Hawkley, L. C., & Cacioppo, J. T. (2010). Loneliness Matters: A Theoretical and Empirical Review of Consequences and Mechanisms. *Annals of Behavioral Medicine, 40*(2), 218-227.

Heinks-Maldonado, T. H.,   Mathalon, D. H., Houde, J. F., Gray, M., Faustman, W. O., & Ford, J. M. (2007). Relationship of Imprecise Corollary Discharge in Schizophrenia to Auditory Hallucinations. *Archives of General Psychiatry, 64*(3), 286.

He, M., Deng, C., & Huang, X. (2013). The Role of Hypothalamic H1 Receptor Antagonism in Antipsychotic-Induced   Weight   Gain. *CNS Drugs, 27*(6), 423-434.

Heresco-Levy, U.,   Javitt, D. C.,   Ermilov, M., Mordel, C., Silipo, G., & Lichtenstein, M. (1999). Efficacy of High-Dose Glycine in the Treatment of Enduring   Negative   Symptoms   of Schizophrenia. *Archives of General Psychiatry, 56*(1), 29.

Herold, C.   (2015).   Neuropsychology, autobiographical memory, and hippocampal volume in "younger" and "older" patients with chronic schizophrenia. *Frontiers in Psychiatry, 6.*

Hertenstein, M. J., Keltner, D., App, B., Bulleit, B. A., & Jaskolka, A. R. (2006). Touch communicates distinct emotions. *Emotion, 6*(3), 528-533.

Holbrook, C., Hahn-Holbrook, J., & Holt-Lunstad, J. (2015). Self-reported spirituality correlates with endogenous oxytocin. *Psychology of Religion and Spirituality, 7*(1), 46-50.

Hong, L. E., Wonodi, I., Lewis, J., & Thaker, G. K.

(2007). Nicotine Effect on Prepulse Inhibition and Prepulse Facilitation in Schizophrenia Patients. *Neuropsychopharmacology, 33*(9), 2167-2174.

Humpston, C. S. (2013). Perplexity and Meaning: Toward a Phenomenological "Core" of Psychotic Experiences. *Schizophrenia Bulletin, 40*(2), 240-243.

Hurd, Y. L., Suzuki, M., & Sedvall, G. C. (2001). D1 and D2 dopamine receptor mRNA expression in whole hemisphere sections of the human brain. *Journal of Chemical Neuroanatomy, 22*(1-2), 127-137.

Imfeld, P., Bodmer, M., Jick, S. S., & Meier, C. R. (2012). Metformin, Other Antidiabetic Drugs, and Risk of Alzheimer's Disease: A Population-Based Case-Control Study. *Journal of the American Geriatrics Society, 60*(5), 916-921.

Jankowski, M., Hajjar, F., Kawas, S. A., Mukaddam-Daher, S., Hoffman, G., McCann, S. M., & Gutkowska, J. (1998). Rat heart: A site of oxytocin production and action. *Proceedings of the National Academy of Sciences, 95*(24), 14558-14563.

Jenkins et al (1984)

Jindal, R. D., Pillai, A. K., Mahadik, S. P., Eklund, K., Montrose, D. M., & Keshavan, M. S. (2010). Decreased BDNF in patients with antipsychotic naïve first episode schizophrenia. *Schizophrenia Research, 119*(1-3), 47-51.

Johnson, N. D., & Mislin, A. (2010). Trust Games: A Meta-Analysis. *SSRN Electronic Journal*.

Jones, H. E., & Griffiths, R. R. (2003). Oral caffeine maintenance potentiates the reinforcing and stimulant subjective effects of intravenous nicotine in cigarette smokers. *Psychopharmacology, 165*(3), 280-290.

Joule, R., & Guéguen, N. (2007). Touch, Compliance, and Awareness of Tactile Contact. *Perceptual and Motor Skills, 104*(2), 581-588.

Jubelt, L. E., Barr, R. S., Goff, D. C., Logvinenko, T., Weiss, A. P., & Evins, A. E. (2008). Effects of transdermal nicotine on episodic memory in non-smokers with and without schizophrenia. *Psychopharmacology, 199*(1), 89-98.

Kane, J. (1988). Clozapine for the Treatment-Resistant Schizophrenic. *Archives of General Psychiatry, 45*(9), 789.

Kapur, S. (2003). Psychosis as a State of Aberrant Salience: A Framework Linking Biology, Phenomenology, and Pharmacology in Schizophrenia. *American Journal of Psychiatry, 160*(1), 13-23.

Kelsch, C. B., Mendez, A. J., Kremer, H., Ironson, G., Schneiderman, N., & Szeto, A. (n.d.). The Relationship of Spirituality, Benefit Finding, and Other Psychosocial Variables to the Hormone Oxytocin in

HIV/AIDS. *Research in the Social Scientific Study of Religion*, 137-162.

King-Casas, B. (2005). Getting to Know You: Reputation and Trust in a Two-Person Economic Exchange. *Science, 308*(5718), 78-83.

Kisely, S., & Campbell, L. A. (2008). Use of Smoking Cessation Therapies in Individuals with Psychiatric Illness. *CNS Drugs, 22*(4), 263-273.

Kjaer, T. W., Bertelsen, C., Piccini, P., Brooks, D., Alving, J., & Lou, H. C. (2002). Increased dopamine tone during meditation-induced change of consciousness. *Cognitive Brain Research, 13*(2), 255-259.

Klein, S. B., Robertson, T. E., & Delton, A. W. (2009). Facing the future: Memory as an evolved system for planning future acts. *Memory & Cognition, 38*(1), 13-22.

Klein, T. A., Endrass, T., Kathmann, N., Neumann, J., Von Cramon, D. Y., & Ullsperger, M. (2007). Neural correlates of error awareness. *NeuroImage, 34*(4), 1774-1781.

Kluge, M., Schuld, A., Himmerich, H., Dalal, M., Schacht, A., Wehmeier, P. M., Hinze-Selch, D., Kraus, T., Dittmann, R. W., & Pollmächer, T. (2007). Clozapine and Olanzapine Are Associated With Food Craving and Binge Eating. *Journal of Clinical Psychopharmacology, 27*(6), 662-666.

Kohls, N., Sauer, S., Offenbacher, M., & Giordano, J.

(2011). Spirituality: an overlooked predictor of placebo effects? *Philosophical Transactions of the Royal Society B: Biological Sciences, 366*(1572), 1838-1848.

Kroeze, W. K., Hufeisen, S. J., Popadak, B. A., Renock, S. M., Steinberg, S., Ernsberger, P., Jayathilake, K., Meltzer, H. Y., & Roth, B. L. (2003). H1-Histamine Receptor Affinity Predicts Short-Term Weight Gain for Typical and Atypical Antipsychotic Drugs. *Neuropsychopharmacology, 28*(3), 519-526.

Larson, C. A., & Carey, K. B. (1998). Caffeine: Brewing trouble in mental health settings? *Professional Psychology: Research and Practice, 29*(4), 373-376.

Lavretsky, H., Zheng, L., Weiner, M. W., Mungas, D., Reed, B., Kramer, J. H., Jagust, W., Chui, H., & Mack, W. J. (2010). Association of Depressed Mood and Mortality in Older Adults With and Without Cognitive Impairment in a Prospective Naturalistic Study. *American Journal of Psychiatry, 167*(5), 589-597.

Lee, K., Farrow, T. F., Spence, S. A., & Woodruff, P. W. (2004). Social cognition, brain networks and schizophrenia. *Psychological Medicine, 34*(3), 391-400.

Lehrer, D. S., & Lorenz, J. (2014). Anosognosia in schizophrenia: Hidden in plain sight. *Innovations in clinical neuroscience, 11*(5-6), 10-17.

Lian, J., Huang, X., Pai, N., & Deng, C. (2014). Betahistine ameliorates olanzapine-induced weight gain through modulation of histaminergic, NPY and

AMPK pathways. *Psychoneuroendocrinology, 48,* 77-86.

Lian, J., Huang, X., Pai, N., & Deng, C. (2016). Ameliorating antipsychotic-induced weight gain by betahistine: Mechanisms and clinical implications. *Pharmacological Research, 106,* 51-63.

Maas, J. W., Bowden, C. L., Miller, A. L., Javors, M. A., Funderburg, L. G., Berman, N., & Weintraub, S. T. (1997). Schizophrenia, Psychosis, and Cerebral Spinal Fluid Homovanillic Acid Concentrations. *Schizophrenia Bulletin, 23*(1), 147-154.

MacKillop, J., & Tidey, J. W. (2011). Cigarette demand and delayed reward discounting in nicotine-dependent individuals with schizophrenia and controls: an initial study. *Psychopharmacology, 216*(1), 91-99.

Mann, J. J. (2003). Neurobiology of suicidal behaviour. *Nature Reviews Neuroscience, 4*(10), 819-828.

Manzella, F. (2015). Smoking in schizophrenic patients: A critique of the self-medication hypothesis. *World Journal of Psychiatry, 5*(1), 35.

Masi, C. M., Chen, H., Hawkley, L. C., & Cacioppo, J. T. (2010). A Meta-Analysis of Interventions to Reduce Loneliness. *Personality and Social Psychology Review, 15*(3), 219-266.

Mather, M., Clewett, D., Sakaki, M., & Harley, C. W. (2015). Norepinephrine ignites local hotspots of neuronal excitation: How arousal amplifies selectivity in perception and memory. *Behavioral and Brain Sciences, 39.*

Mazure, C. M., Nelson, J., Jatlow, P. I., & Bowers, M. B. (1991). Plasma free homovanillic acid (HVA) as a predictor of clinical response in acute psychosis. *Biological Psychiatry, 30*(5), 475-482.

McGuire, P., Howes, O., Stone, J., & Fusarpoli, P. (2008). Functional neuroimaging in schizophrenia: diagnosis and drug discovery. *Trends in Pharmacological Sciences, 29*(2), 91-98.

Meltzoff, A., & Moore, M. (1977). Imitation of facial and manual gestures by human neonates. *Science, 198*(4312), 74-78.

Meskanen, K., Ekelund, H., Laitinen, J., Neuvonen, P. J., Haukka, J., Panula, P., & Ekelund, J. (2013). A Randomized Clinical Trial of Histamine 2 Receptor Antagonism in Treatment-Resistant Schizophrenia. *Journal of Clinical Psychopharmacology, 33*(4), 472-478.

Modinos, G., Costafreda, S. G., Van Tol, M., McGuire, P. K., Aleman, A., & Allen, P. (2013). Neuroanatomy of auditory verbal hallucinations in schizophrenia: A quantitative meta-analysis of voxel-based morphometry studies. *Cortex, 49*(4), 1046-1055.

Mohandas, E. (2008). Neurobiology of

Spirituality. *Mens Sana Monographs, 6*(1), 63.

Mohr, W. K. (2006). Spiritual Issues in Psychiatric Care. *Perspectives In Psychiatric Care, 42*(3), 174-183.

Molteni, R., Barnard, R., Ying, Z., Roberts, C., & Gómez-Pinilla, F. (2002). A high-fat, refined sugar diet reduces hippocampal brain-derived neurotrophic factor, neuronal plasticity, and learning. *Neuroscience, 112*(4), 803-814.

Moore, E., Mander, A., Ames, D., Kotowicz, M., Carne, R., Brodaty, H., Woodward, M., et al.(2013). Increased risk of cognitive impairment in patients with diabetes is associated with metformin. Diabetes Care 2013;36:2981-2987. *Diabetes Care, 36*(11), 3850-3850.

Moretto, G., Sellitto, M., & Di Pellegrino, G. (2013). Investment and repayment in a trust game after ventromedial prefrontal damage. *Frontiers in Human Neuroscience, 7.*

Mulert, C., Kirsch, V., Pascual-Marqui, R., McCarley, R. W., & Spencer, K. M. (2011). Long-range synchrony of gamma oscillations and auditory hallucination symptoms in schizophrenia. *International Journal of Psychophysiology, 79*(1), 55-63.

Nakama, H., Chang, L., Fein, G., Shimotsu, R., Jiang, C. S., & Ernst, T. (2011). Methamphetamine users show greater than normal age-related cortical gray matter loss. *Addiction, 106*(8), 1474-1483.

Naqvi, N. H., & Bechara, A. (2009). The hidden island of addiction: the insula. *Trends in Neurosciences, 32*(1), 56-67.

Nelson, M. D., Saykin, A. J., Flashman, L. A., & Riordan, H. J. (1997). Hippocampal volume reduction in schizophrenia as assessed by magnetic resonance imaging: A meta-analytic study. *Schizophrenia Research, 24*(1-2), 153.

Ng, T. P., Feng, L., Yap, K. B., Lee, T. S., Tan, C. H., & Winblad, B. (2014). Long-Term Metformin Usage and Cognitive Function among Older Adults with Diabetes. *Journal of Alzheimer's Disease, 41*(1), 61-68.

Nummenmaa, L., Tuominen, L., Dunbar, R., Hirvonen, J., Manninen, S., Arponen, E., Machin, A., Hari, R., Jaaskelainen, I. P., & Sams, M. (2016). Social touch modulates endogenous μ-opioid system activity in humans. *Neuroimage, 138*, 242-247.

Ohlsson, B., Truedsson, M., Djerf, P., & Sundler, F. (2006). Oxytocin is expressed throughout the human gastrointestinal tract. *Regulatory Peptides, 135*(1-2), 7-11.

Palaniyappan, L., Mallikarjun, P., Joseph, V., White, T. P., & Liddle, P. F. (2010). Reality distortion is related to the structure of the salience network in schizophrenia. *Psychological Medicine, 41*(08), 1701-1708.

Palaniyappan, L. (2012). Does the salience network play a cardinal role in psychosis? An emerging hypothesis of insular dysfunction. *Journal of Psychiatry & Neuroscience, 37*(1), 17-27.

Pantelis, C. (2005). Structural Brain Imaging Evidence for Multiple Pathological Processes at Different Stages of Brain Development in Schizophrenia. *Schizophrenia Bulletin, 31*(3), 672-696.

Parikh, V., Kutlu, M. G., & Gould, T. J. (2016). nAChR dysfunction as a common substrate for schizophrenia and comorbid nicotine addiction: Current trends and perspectives. *Schizophrenia Research, 171*(1-3), 1-15.

Parikh, V., Kutlu, M. G., & Gould, T. J. (2016). nAChR dysfunction as a common substrate for schizophrenia and comorbid nicotine addiction: Current trends and perspectives. *Schizophrenia Research, 171*(1-3), 1-15.

Paska, A. V., Zupanc, T., & Pregelj, P. (2013). The role of brain-derived neurotrophic factor in the pathophysiology of suicidal behavior. *Psychiatria Danubina, 25*(2), 341-344.

Peciña, S., Smith, K. S., & Berridge, K. C. (2006). Hedonic Hot Spots in the Brain. *The Neuroscientist, 12*(6), 500-511.

Peet, M. (2004). Nutrition and schizophrenia: beyond omega-3 fatty acids. *Prostaglandins, Leukotrienes and Essential Fatty Acids, 70*(4), 417-422.

Pickar, D., Labarca, R., Linnoila, M., Roy, A., Hommer, D., Everett, D., & Paul, S. (1984). Neuroleptic-induced decrease in plasma homovanillic acid and antipsychotic activity in schizophrenic patients. *Science, 225*(4665), 954-957.

Piedmont, R. L. (1999). Does Spirituality Represent the Sixth Factor of Personality? Spiritual Transcendence and the Five-Factor Model. *Journal of Personality, 67*(6), 985-1013.

Pontieri, F. E., Tanda, G., Orzi, F., & Chiara, G. D. (1996). Effects of nicotine on the nucleus accumbens and similarity to those of addictive drugs. *Nature, 382*(6588), 255-257.

Potts, M., & Lim, D. (2012). An Old Drug for New Ideas: Metformin Promotes Adult Neurogenesis and Spatial Memory Formation. *Cell Stem Cell, 11*(1), 5-6.

Poyurovsky, M., Pashinian, A., Levi, A., Weizman, R., & Weizman, A. (2005). The effect of betahistine, a histamine H1 receptor agonist/H3 antagonist, on olanzapine-induced weight gain in first-episode schizophrenia patients. *International Clinical Psychopharmacology, 20*(2), 101-103.

Prochaska, J. J. (2010). Failure to treat tobacco use in mental health and addiction treatment settings: A form of harm reduction? *Drug and Alcohol Dependence, 110*(3), 177-182.

Ribeiro, J. A., & Sebastião, A. M. (2010). Caffeine and Adenosine. *Journal of Alzheimer's Disease*, 20(s1), S3-S15.

Rizos, E., Papathanasiou, M., Michalopoulou, P., Mazioti, A., Douzenis, A., Kastania, A., Nikolaidou, P., Laskos, E., Vasilopoulou, K., & Lykouras, L. (2011). Association of serum BDNF levels with hippocampal volumes in first psychotic episode drug-naive schizophrenic patients. *Schizophrenia Research, 129*(2-3), 201-204.

Rizos, E., Papathanasiou, M. A., Michalopoulou, P. G., Laskos, E., Mazioti, A., Kastania, A., Vasilopoulou, K.,. et al. (2014). A Longitudinal Study of Alterations of Hippocampal Volumes and Serum BDNF Levels in Association to Atypical Antipsychotics in a Sample of First-Episode Patients with Schizophrenia. *PLoS ONE, 9*(2), e87997.

Rosenfeld, A. J., Lieberman, J. A., & Jarskog, L. F. (2010). Oxytocin, Dopamine, and the Amygdala: A Neurofunctional Model of Social Cognitive Deficits in Schizophrenia. *Schizophrenia Bulletin, 37*(5), 1077-1087.

Sagud, M., Mihaljevic-Peles, A., Muck-Seler, D., Pivac, N., Vuksan-Cusa, B., Brataljenovic, T., & Jakovljevic, M. (2009). Smoking and Schizophrenia. *Psychiatria Danubina, 21*(3), 371-375.

Sahu, G., Malavade, K., & Jacob, T. (2015). Cognitive Impairment in Schizophrenia: Interplay of BDNF and Childhood Trauma? A Review of

Literature. *Psychiatric Quarterly, 87*(3), 559-569.

Sapolsky, R. M. (2000). The possibility of neurotoxicity in the hippocampus in major depression: a primer on neuron death. *Biological Psychiatry, 48*(8), 755-765.

Schjoedt, U. (2009). The Religious Brain: A General Introduction to the Experimental Neuroscience of Religion. *Method & Theory in the Study of Religion, 21*(3), 310-339.

SEIDLER, G. H., & WAGNER, F. E. (2006). Comparing the efficacy of EMDR and trauma-focused cognitive-behavioral therapy in the treatment of PTSD: a meta-analytic study. *Psychological Medicine, 36*(11), 1515.

Seidman, L. J., Faraone, S. V., Goldstein, J. M., Goodman, J. M., Kremen, W. S., Toomey, R., Tourville, J., et al. (1999). Thalamic and amygdala–hippocampal volume reductions in first-degree relatives of patients with schizophrenia: an MRI-based morphometric analysis. *Biological Psychiatry, 46*(7), 941-954.

Shalvi, S., & De Dreu, C. K. (2014). Oxytocin promotes group-serving dishonesty. *Proceedings of the National Academy of Sciences, 111*(15), 5503-5507.

Shapiro, F. (2014). The Role of Eye Movement Desensitization and Reprocessing (EMDR) Therapy in Medicine: Addressing the Psychological and Physical

Symptoms Stemming from Adverse Life Experience. *The Permanente Journal*, 71-77.

Shariff, M., Quik, M., Holgate, J., Morgan, M., Patkar, O. L., Tam, V., Belmer, A., & Bartlett, S. E. (2016). Neuronal Nicotinic Acetylcholine Receptor Modulators Reduce Sugar Intake. *PLOS ONE, 11*(3), e0150270.

Sher, L. (2010). Brain-derived neurotrophic factor and suicidal behavior. *QJM, 104*(5), 455-458.

Smith, G. N., Wong, H., MacEwan, G. W., Kopala, L. C., Ehmann, T. S., Thornton, A. E., Lang, D. J., et al. (2009). Predictors of starting to smoke cigarettes in patients with first episode psychosis. *Schizophrenia Research, 108*(1-3), 258-264.

Thomas, N., Ravan, J., Jebaraj, P., & Braganza, D. (2009). Clozapine producing weight loss: A case series with possible clinical implications - A hypothesis. *Journal of Postgraduate Medicine, 55*(4), 317.

Thompson, L., Pennay, A., Zimmermann, A., Cox, M., & Lubman, D. I. (2014). "Clozapine makes me quite drowsy, so when I wake up in the morning those first cups of coffee are really handy": an exploratory qualitative study of excessive caffeine consumption among individuals with schizophrenia. *BMC Psychiatry, 14*(1).

Tiwari, S. (2013). Loneliness: A disease? *Indian Journal of Psychiatry, 55*(4), 320.

Tormey, W., Carney, M., & FitzGerald, R. (1999). Catecholamines in urine after death. *Forensic Science International, 103*(1), 67-71.

Tungaraza, T. E. (2016). Significant weight loss following clozapine use, how is it possible? A case report and review of published cases and literature relevant to the subject. *Therapeutic Advances in Psychopharmacology, 6*(5), 335-342.

Uhlhaas, P., Roux, F., & Singer, W. (2011). S.19.04 The role of oscillations and synchrony in cortical networks and their putative relevance for the pathophysiology of schizophrenia. *European Neuropsychopharmacology, 21*, S217.

Uhlhaas, P. J., & Singer, W. (2010). Abnormal neural oscillations and synchrony in schizophrenia. *Nature Reviews Neuroscience, 11*(2), 100-113.

Van Cappellen, P., Way, B. M., Isgett, S. F., & Fredrickson, B. L. (2016). Effects of oxytocin administration on spirituality and emotional responses to meditation. *Social Cognitive and Affective Neuroscience, 11*(10), 1579-1587.

Van IJzendoorn, M. H., & Bakermans-Kranenburg, M. J. (2012). A sniff of trust: Meta-analysis of the effects of intranasal oxytocin administration on face recognition, trust to in-group, and trust to out-group. *Psychoneuroendocrinology, 37*(3), 438-443.

Vysata, O., Kukal, J., Prochazka, A., Pazdera, L., Simko, J., & Valis, M. (2014). Age-related changes in EEG coherence. *Neurologia i Neurochirurgia Polska, 48*(1), 35-38.

Weickert, C. S., Hyde, T. M., Lipska, B. K., Herman, M. M., Weinberger, D. R., & Kleinman, J. E. (2003). Reduced brain-derived neurotrophic factor in prefrontal cortex of patients with schizophrenia. *Molecular Psychiatry, 8*(6), 592-610.

Whitcher, S. J., & Fisher, J. D. (1979). Multidimensional reaction to therapeutic touch in a hospital setting. *Journal of Personality and Social Psychology, 37*(1), 87-96.

White, T. P., Joseph, V., Francis, S. T., & Liddle, P. F. (2010, November). Aberrant salience network (bilateral insula and anterior cingulate cortex) connectivity during information processing in schizophrenia. *Schizophrenia Research, 123*(2-3), 105-115.

Wong, D., Wagner, H., Tune, L., Dannals, R., Pearlson, G., Links, J., Tamminga, C., et al. (1986). Positron emission tomography reveals elevated D2 dopamine receptors in drug-naive schizophrenics. *Science, 234*(4783), 1558-1563.

Wylie, K. P., & Tregellas, J. R. (2010). The role of the insula in schizophrenia. *Schizophrenia Research, 123*(2-3), 93-104.

Xu, F., Plummer, M. R., Len, G., Nakazawa, T., Yamamoto, T., Black, I. B., & Wu, K. (2006). Brain-derived neurotrophic factor rapidly increases NMDA receptor channel activity through Fyn-mediated phosphorylation. *Brain Research, 1121*(1), 22-34.

Yaden, D. B., Iwry, J., & Newberg, A. B. (2017). Neuroscience and religion: surveying the field. In *Religion: Mental Religion* (pp. 277-299). Macmillan Reference.

Zimmermann, A., Lubman, D. I., & Cox, M. (2012). Tobacco, Caffeine, Alcohol and Illicit Substance Use Among Consumers of a National Psychiatric Disability Support Service. *International Journal of Mental Health and Addiction, 10*(5), 722-736.

Zimmermann, A., Lubman, D. I., & Cox, M. (2012). Tobacco, caffeine, alcohol and illicit substance use among consumers of a national community managed mental health service. *Mental Health and Substance Use, 5*(4), 287-302.

Zipursky, R. B., Reilly, T. J., & Murray, R. M. (2012). The Myth of Schizophrenia as a Progressive Brain Disease. *Schizophrenia Bulletin, 39*(6), 1363-1372.

www.ingramcontent.com/pod-product-compliance
Lightning Source LLC
Chambersburg PA
CBHW062203270326
41930CB00009B/1633